Caesarean

About one quarter of births across the UK, Europe and the USA are now by caesarean and the debate provoked by the steadily escalating rates invariably produces more heat than light. The multitude of interested parties – midwives, obstetricians, parents, activists and managers – means that the many different groups talk at cross purposes and without listening to each other.

Through this controversial book, Rosemary Mander, a practising midwife and researcher, seeks to find the meaning of caesarean. It critically analyses the place of caesarean in contemporary childbearing and questions the changes that are taking place in childbirth. It explores, in particular, the effects and implications of the increase in caesarean births, and includes discussion of:

- the context of the operation and repercussions
- caesarean rates around the world and their relation to health systems
- decision making and cultural/medical constraints
- the short- and long-term implications of caesarean for the woman and her baby.

Using a strong research evidence base, Rosemary Mander concludes that the caesarean may not necessarily benefit either the woman or her baby. Rather, it may benefit those professionals whose investment is in extending the range of their influence.

Caesarean is accessible to a range of readers and will be of particular interest to the health care provider and the childbearing woman.

Rosemary Mander is Professor of Midwifery at the University of Edinburgh, Scotland. She is both a practising midwife and an active midwifery researcher.

Caesarean

Just another way of birth?

Rosemary Mander

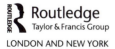

Routledge
Taylor & Francis Group

LONDON AND NEW YORK

First published 2007 by Routledge
2 Park Square, Milton Park, Abingdon, Oxon OX14 4RN

Simultaneously published in the USA and Canada
by Routledge
270 Madison Ave, New York, NY 10016

Routledge is an imprint of the Taylor & Francis Group, an informa business

© 2007 Rosemary Mander

Typeset in Times by
Keystroke, 28 High Street, Tettenhall, Wolverhampton
Printed and bound in Great Britain by
Antony Rowe Ltd, Chippenham, Wiltshire

British Library Cataloguing in Publication Data
A catalogue record for this book is available from the British Library

Library of Congress Cataloging in Publication Data
A catalog record for this book has been requested

ISBN10: 0–415–40135–6 (hbk)
ISBN10: 0–415–40136–4 (pbk)
ISBN10: 0–203–96076–9 (ebk)

ISBN13: 978–0–415–40135–7 (hbk)
ISBN13: 978–0–415–40136–4 (pbk)
ISBN13: 978–0–203–96076–9 (ebk)

Contents

Acknowledgements

I acknowledge the inspiration of the women and the midwives with whom I have had the privilege to practise. I have learned more from them than they will ever realise.

Although this book is my responsibility, I would like to thank the following for sharing their thoughts, their ideas and sometimes their work with me: Agency for Healthcare Research and Policy, Alison MacFarlane, Beverley L. Beech, Chryssoula Lemonidou, David Lamb, Debbie Harrison, Deborah Purdue, Ekaterini Kasidi, Elias Mossialos, Geraldine Barrett, Gian Carlo DiRenzo, Gordon Lyons, Graeme D. Smith, Irena A. Frei, Irene Calvert, Jackie Baxter, Jane Weaver, Jenny Newland, Kath Melia, National Childbirth Trust, Ngai Fen Cheung, Norelle Groeschel, RCM Library, Sheila Kitzinger, Sarah Stewart, Sinead McNally, Steve Tilley and Wang Liston.

My most profound thanks go to Iain Abbot. His searching questions, while not always welcomed, may have enhanced the material in the book.

Introduction

There is considerable media interest in the caesarean operation. This interest is found not only in the professional, but also the popular media. The public interest is not due to the generally increasing numbers of babies born by this route. The interest is more in the media celebrities who choose to give birth by caesarean. While an interest in childbearing among 'celebs' may be understandable, we must bear in mind that this interest does not reflect an interest in the operation *per se*, but merely a general preoccupation with media personalities.

The debate on caesarean invariably engenders more heat than light. The multitude of interested parties, or stakeholders, means that the many different interest groups tend to talk at cross-purposes, that is, without paying attention to each other. It is my intention that this book should address the wide range of issues which these interest groups would raise. The hope is that it will stimulate a constructive dialogue between all of the interested parties. The important issues relating to caesarean are the concern of not just those who undergo these operations, nor just those who are involved with performing them. The issues raised by caesarean affect a large section of society and a large proportion of its members. This book aims to show how these wide-ranging effects happen and to discuss their likely implications.

Throughout this book I seek to support my arguments by reference to the relevant research as well as other literature. While I endeavour to make this approach as reader-friendly as possible, some may find that the inclusion of references in the text is a distraction. These references matter, though. This is because they serve to support my argument and they also demonstrate the currency or historical nature of the sources. I would advise readers who may be less than accustomed to this style of writing to regard the references not as a distraction, but as a further source of helpful information.

It may then be helpful to the reader for me to explain my personal interest in caesarean. My ongoing personal experience as a midwife has undoubtedly influenced my interpretation of the meaning of caesarean. To this personal experience, though, must be added my experience of teaching and undertaking research in an institution of higher education. Crucial to this latter experience has been the need to question certain generally accepted aspects of maternity care. Such experience and questioning, I consider, enables me to adopt a more complete understanding and to provide a more holistic picture of the phenomenon which is caesarean. If some readers consider that my background may have resulted in a critical, a negative or even a feminist-leaning orientation, I certainly do not regard this as a problem.

My experience and questioning has led me to adopt a certain view of caesarean, which will emerge through the medium of this book. This view may be perceived as unevenly balanced. Balanced views, though, are more likely to be reached by some compromise of sources. It may be unfortunate that stringent analysis of research-based material is unlikely to lead to the balance which some may seek.

Further, my view of caesarean may be criticised on the grounds that it may be unhelpful to women; especially the woman who has experienced a caesarean and who may not be entirely happy with her experience. Such women's feelings, I suspect, are so deeply ingrained that they are not likely to be affected by what is said or written by others, regardless of the basis of those sayings or writings. There are, of course, those professionals and experts who may be concerned that this approach is not suitable for childbearing women. I venture to suggest that these women are not stupid and should not be treated patronisingly. Such women require factual research-based information and certainly not euphemisms, half-truths or unfounded assumptions.

Thus, for these reasons I contend that the material in this book is *per se* neither harmful nor dangerous. It may be that the reverse applies, in that a consistently argued rationale may provide illumination to light some of the darker corners of such women's experiences.

The argument advanced by this book develops progressively through the nine chapters. The book opens with a backwards glance which shows how the caesarean operation has evolved from being a way of avoiding an unacceptable outcome into a highly desired birthing option. This background then widens its focus to consider why this intervention is so significant. In Chapter 2, I probe the crucial role of research in this particular aspect of maternity care. Chapter 3 adopts an evidence-based approach to examine the debates which rage around the various aspects of the actual surgical operation. This chapter illuminates a number of important issues relating to decision making in health care. The globalisation of health care is recognised in Chapter 4 to demonstrate the significance of caesarean on the international stage. The various factors which influence the international picture are teased out in order to show their relative importance in the differing settings. One of these various factors is the culture of childbearing which, in turn, determines the focus in Chapter 5 on decision making. This focus takes in the relationships between service providers and users and between the occupational groups involved in maternity care. In Chapters 6 and 7 the health and other implications of caesarean are addressed. This includes examinations of, first, the short-term and then the long-term effects. The eighth chapter seeks to explore one of the means which have been widely recommended to reduce the numbers of caesareans. This material shows the limited extent to which research evidence is utilised in obstetric practice.

The book concludes by revisiting the status of the caesarean and an analysis of its ultimate or longest of long-term implications. The conclusion emerges that the benefits of this surgical operation may accrue to someone other than the woman or 'patient' on whom the caesarean is performed or to the baby or babies who are birthed by this surgical intervention.

In order to complete the Introduction to this book and this topic, I would like to mention a phrase which clearly demonstrates the disconcerting nature of the caesarean operation. It has very appropriately been referred to as the 'mother of all interventions' (Stapleton, 2004:103). The term is associated with the phrase made notorious by Saddam Hussein in 1991. He was referring to the military preparations for the Gulf War which would constitute 'The mother of all battles'. This phrase has come to represent a misplaced confidence of a successful outcome to some form of struggle. It is necessary to reflect on Stapleton's use of this phrase. The reader is left to wonder to which struggle she was referring. It may be too early to decide whether this phrase was a prediction or merely wishful thinking.

1 'The game of the name'

Like the origins of the operation itself, the origins of the name 'caesarean' are obscure. In an attempt to introduce this all-too-familiar intervention in childbearing, I focus, first, on the word and how it and the operation originally came to be used. I then seek to address the significance of caesarean. This is initially in numerical terms, but it is also necessary to relate caesarean, most importantly, to 'normal childbearing' and, then, to intervention in childbearing. I argue that the name which this operation was given may have been crucial to its eventual widespread acceptance.

1 BEGINNINGS

The origins of the caesarean are so shrouded in the mists of myth that speculation is not uncommonly presented as fact. In order to disentangle the mythology from more verifiable reality, I approach the origins by differentiating the words used from the history of the operation. While the history, or versions of it, is relatively well-known, the words have passed into common usage, apparently bypassing any thought processes. Although this distinction between words and deeds may appear artificial, I would argue that there is much to learn from both.

1.1 Terminology

I have borrowed the title of this chapter from Sheahan, who used this phrase to examine the meanings of the term 'nurse' (1972). In the same way, the name given to this operation speaks volumes about how it is perceived. Further, the variations in terminology to describe the caesarean demonstrate the variety of interested parties. I attempt here to address the terminology and then justify my rationale for using the term 'caesarean'.

Before focusing on the word itself, though, I would like to offer a definition in order to clarify the nature of this phenomenon. The caesarean is nothing more or less than the delivery of a viable baby (or babies) via a surgical incision through the muscular wall of the mother's uterus or womb and the layers which make up the wall of her abdomen. The viability of the baby matters, because an operation before the baby is considered viable would constitute a termination of pregnancy or hysterotomy. In the UK at the time of writing the lower limit of viability is twenty-four weeks' gestation. The definition which I have offered is useful because there are no assumptions about the 'intendedness', the indications for, or the circumstances of the delivery; I use the word 'delivery' advisedly here, because of the woman usually being quite passive during the actual operation.

The word's origins relate to their study, or etymology, which, in the medieval world, was crucial to substantiating theory (Blumenfeld-Kosinski, 1990:143). The identification, or possibly the creation, of etymological links was used to lend authority to otherwise spurious claims to veracity. It was in this slightly questionable intellectual environment that 'legendary and medical material coalesced' (1990:144) to bequeath to us the legacy of the myth of Gaius Julius Caesar's birth in 100 BCE (see below).

The word 'caesarean' is more likely, though, to derive from the *lex regia* (royal law), which had been introduced in the eighth century BCE (Blumenfeld-Kosinski, 1990:145). This legislation required that the baby of a woman dying undelivered should be removed surgically, because the burial of a pregnant woman was expressly forbidden. The rationale for this intervention may be explained in terms of an attempt to, at least, rescue the baby (Lurie, 2005). Trolle, though, is less certain. He argues persuasively that an alternative reason would be to prevent the gruesomely unacceptable possibility of a post-mortem spontaneous birth (1982:16) or 'coffin birth' (Boyd, 2003). This disconcerting phenomenon may take place a couple of days or more after the pregnant woman's death, as a result of the increasing pressure of gases resulting from putrefaction.

The *lex regia* subsequently became known as the *lex caesarea*, due to *caeso matris utero* (to cut from the mother's uterus). Children born by this route were dubbed *caesones* (Trolle, 1982:25). As de Costa points out, Julius was not a *caesone*, but he was one in a long line to bear the name 'Caesar'. She adds that probably one of his ancestors had been born in this way and that 'the man was named from the operation, rather than the reverse' (2001:97). There are, additionally, a number of alternative explanations of the origin of the name, which may relate to hairiness, eye colour or hunting prowess (Trolle, 1982:25).

During the first millennium, surgical skills and interest in Julius Caesar developed alongside each other. The name 'caesarean', however, was not actually applied to this surgical operation until François Rousset in France in 1581 used the tautologous phrase, '*section caesarienne*' (Blumenfeld-Kosinski, 1990:153; Trolle, 1982:28). This term, because of the fashionable hagiography of Julius Caesar, was accepted and soon spread widely. The English version appeared in a translation of Guillemeau's textbook in 1612. Since that time, presumably in honour of the supposedly eponymous hero, an uppercase initial has often been used. This persists, despite the general acceptance of the mythical nature of the link with Gaius Julius Caesar. Similarly mistakenly, the spelling 'Caesarian' is defined as 'of or relating to or in the manner of Julius Caesar' (Princeton, 2005).

The mythical link between the operation and the Roman emperor Gaius Julius Caesar is further clarified by a brief examination of another language's terminology.

In the various forms of the German language the operation is consistently referred to colloquially as '*der Kaiserschnitt*' (Frei, 2005; Quecke, 1952). Literally translated, this means 'the emperor cut'. Whether the emperor in question is Gaius Julius Caesar is not known. The fact that people in German-speaking countries, however, invariably refer to this person as 'Kaiser Julius Caesar' suggests that 'der Kaiserschnitt' could relate to any emperor.

In the latter part of the twentieth century, though, in association with the globalisation of obstetrics and the medicalisation of childbearing, new terms became more prevalent. Due mainly to the frequency of this operation's use on the other side of the Atlantic, the terms 'cesarean' and 'c-section' have become commonplace. Particularly insidious, though, is the abbreviation of the generally accepted caesarean/cesarean section simply to 'section': 'I had an emergency section with [name of baby] after a prolonged latent phase' (Helen, 2004).

The term 'section', and possibly 'caesarean section', serves to trivialise this major abdominal surgery, because 'section' means nothing more than 'cut' (Oakley, 1983). These terms have been accepted into general usage, as shown in Helen's words from a website (above). These changes in the words have reduced perceptions of the seriousness of this operation and its inherent risks (please see Chapters 6 and 7). Again, the influence of the North American health care systems may be held responsible. The result is that caesarean is trivialised to such an extent that it is now widely accepted as little more than just another form of birth. For this reason the terms 'caesarean', 'caesarean operation' or 'caesarean procedure' are more appropriate and are the words that I use in this book.

While considering the terminology used here, I should mention that, in this book, I write about the 'baby', irrespective of how many are involved. This is to avoid clumsy devices, such as 'baby/babies'.

1.2 History

The discussion of the origins of the word 'caesarean' has given us some clues as to the history of the operation. While I now focus on that history, it is necessary to look, first, at the operation's fabulous associations. Like Trolle (1982), in order to be faithful to the literature, I avoid using the word 'caesarean' for any operation before 1581, when Rousset introduced it. It is necessary to recognise, though, that much of the information available about the history of caesarean is inaccurate to the point of myth (NTUH, 2005; Sehdev, 2005).

1.2.1 Legend and myth and fiction

As I have suggested already, the origins of the abdominal delivery extend beyond history into the realms of mythology. Whether it is possible to disentangle history from mythology is not yet certain. Perhaps because of the innate humanness of giving birth vaginally, the alternative abdominal birth has featured frequently and prominently in the myths and legends of the births of deities. Trolle explains this phenomenon in terms of abdominal birth being 'the godly way to enter the world'

(1982:9). The Greek gods who arrived by this route include Zeus delivering Dionysus, Apollo delivering Aesculapius and the delivery of Adonis. Brahma and Buddha, in eastern mythology, were born in the same way. Abdominal birth also figures in Roman, Persian, Icelandic, Irish and Danish legends. Perhaps significantly, a number of military heroes have been credited with caesarean birth, including Scipio Africanus, who defeated Hannibal, and Rustam a Persian hero (Lurie, 2005).

It is hardly surprising, therefore, that myths about such a hero as Julius Caesar being delivered abdominally were so easily accepted. That they are myths is evidenced by the fact that at the time of his birth in 100 BCE, abdominal delivery was only performed as a post-mortem operation. Caesar's mother survived his birth by many years, which is demonstrated by his campaign letters to her. Thus, Julius Caesar could not have been born abdominally.

The benefits, or at least the claims to benefit, of caesarean birth were widely recognised as early as the eighteenth century in England. These heroes born in this way are rehearsed by Tristram Shandy's fictional father as he seeks to persuade his pregnant wife to submit herself to the surgeon's knife: 'These, and many more who figured high in the annals of fame,—all came side-way, Sir, into the world' (Sterne, 1769:Chapter 19).

Scottish heroic legends include the story of Marjory Bruce, the only daughter of King Robert the Bruce. After a hunting accident in which she was mortally injured, her son was delivered abdominally and went on to become King Robert II. It may be that this story is the basis of Shakespeare's familiar plot, which features Macduff, who was not 'of woman born', prevailing against Macbeth:

> And let the angel whom thou still has served
> Tell thee, Macduff was from his mother's womb
> Untimely ripp'd.
> (Shakespeare, *Macbeth*, Act V, sc 8.14–16)

So, Shakespeare, like others, represents caesarean as imbuing the person who is born in this way with superhuman powers. The experience of Marjory Bruce may serve to qualify the nature of caesarean as originating as only performed post mortem. Because knowledge of physiology was less well developed, the diagnosis of death may have been less precise. Thus, the operation could have been performed when the woman was either dead or moribund.

1.2.2 The post-mortem operation

The relationship between abdominal delivery and the child developing extraordinary powers occurs too frequently to be ignored. This may be associated with the early Roman legislation, mentioned already, which meant that the operation was invariably performed post mortem. This association may involve the child assuming the spirit of their dying mother or, more prosaically, the need for the motherless child to be extraordinarily talented in order to survive and prosper. Such attributes have been recognised since Pliny the Elder (23–79 CE) wrote in his 'Natural History': 'It is a better omen when the mother dies in giving birth to the child'.

The precise date of the first abdominal delivery is difficult to assess, but the ancient Egyptians are likely to have had the skills to perform the post-mortem operation (Trolle, 1982). Further, there is evidence that the ancient Greeks had also developed these skills by the fourth century BCE, as did the Jews in the second century BCE and, of course, the Romans.

The absence of this operation from any extant literature may be due to physicians' unwillingness to involve themselves with the low status and potentially polluting work of attending the dead (Trolle, 1982:17). This unwillingness is likely to have been aggravated by the traditionally low status and equally polluting attendance at childbirth. In addition, as Trolle suggests, the physician is more than likely to make himself scarce if death is likely to be the outcome (1982:17)

Although we may assume that abdominal delivery has traditionally been the ultimate 'rescue operation', there is the suggestion (above) that this may not have been the case. Regardless of the rationale, it is not possible to be certain of the reality of this 'rescue operation' until the Christian church gave the matter its attention. This did not happen until Thomas Aquinas (1225–74) proposed the need for the newborn to be baptised, in order for the soul to achieve eternal life. In this way, the Christian church presented the physician with a role in childbirth and abdominal delivery appeared in the literature in the early fourteenth century. The Council of Trent (1545–63) reaffirmed, through its emphasis on the fundamentality of the sacraments, the importance of the operation that had still to become known as caesarean.

In considering the post-mortem nature of abdominal delivery, I have made the assumption that it was undertaken if the woman was moribund or had actually expired. It is obvious that the baby *might* survive this operation; King Robert II being but one example. Another royal example of a baby surviving a caesarean was Edward, the son of Jane Seymour and Henry VIII of England. In 1537 his mother survived for eleven days after the birth of the baby who, albeit briefly, became Edward VI. Clearly abdominal delivery had developed into a post-mortem rescue operation. It may be that the woman may not have been actually dead when the operation was begun, but it would be extremely likely that she would be dead by the time the baby was born. These two reasonably well-authenticated examples, however, show that only relatively recently did the baby have a chance of surviving.

Eventually the operation began to be used on the living woman, but this happened only gradually and, to some extent, reluctantly. The Scottish obstetrician William Smellie articulated this reluctance: 'It is better to have recourse to an operation which hath sometimes succeeded than to leave [the woman and baby] to an untimely death' (1752:380–4).

The transition from caesarean being a post-mortem operation to one being performed with some hope of maternal, and possibly fetal, survival caused it to become an emergency operation. This means that it would be performed in labour when, particularly, the mother's life was at risk (Ryan, 2002:462). It was not until much more recently that the possibility of caesarean becoming an elective, that is a planned, intervention materialised.

1.2.3 The caesarean operation on a living woman

The words of the Talmud suggest that Jews, who may not have been surgeons, performed abdominal deliveries in 500 CE, and that the women were alive and survived. Firm evidence, however, is lacking. Similarly, early accounts of operations performed by a lay person or by the woman herself may provide a less than complete picture (Trolle, 1982:29).

Particularly notable or notorious, though, is the tale of Jacob Nufer, a sow gelder in Switzerland at the turn of the sixteenth century. He reputedly ended his wife's prolonged labour by applying his gelding knife to her abdomen. The mother and baby were healthy, so much so that she enjoyed several more successful and physiological pregnancies. That this operation was not reported until ninety-one years later must call into question its veracity. Even if true, however, the ease of the operation and Frau Nufer's subsequent childbearing career suggest that this operation was not actually a caesarean. These factors point to the pregnancy having been situated in the abdominal cavity rather than the uterus (Ainsworth, 2003). This means that, according to the above definition, this could not have been a caesarean, even if the word had been in use at the time. Other examples of 'untrained' people performing abdominal deliveries figure prominently in the literature, suggesting that this operation is not a uniquely medical intervention.

As well as deliberate operations, traumatic abdominal deliveries have been reported (Trolle, 1982:32). Such deliveries feature surprisingly low mortality rates, presumably because of the healthy fetal and maternal condition at the time of the accident.

1.2.4 Factors influencing the historical use of caesarean

As mentioned already the caesarean gradually came to be performed by experienced and/or trained personnel on women who were neither dead nor dying. Surgeons were most likely to perform the operation, although midwives occasionally did so. The poor outcomes (see below), particularly for the mother, gave rise to serious debates about the precedence of maternal life or infant life in emergency situations. These debates resulted in the very different attitudes to caesarean on either side of the English Channel. Whereas the French would be prepared to risk sacrificing the mother in the interests of the survival of the baby, the British were much more reticent about the use of this seriously life-threatening intervention (Churchill, 2003). Although European authors are rather coy about suggesting the influence of religious orientation on historical enthusiasm for the caesarean operation, in America the religious debate was quite explicit (Ryan, 2002). The condition of the mother's and the baby's eternal soul, though, may have had more than a little influence on caesarean decisions.

The most common scenario in which caesarean would be considered would be if the mother and baby were both alive and labour had become obstructed. A frequent cause of obstruction would be cephalo-pelvic disproportion associated with contracted pelvis (de Costa, 2001:98) due to disease, such as childhood rickets (Ryan, 2002). In such a scenario, the alternatives to either caesarean or maternal death included a range of, to modern minds, repugnant interventions. The first group of which became known euphemistically as 'destructive operations' (Garrey et al, 1969:454). These included:

1   Craniotomy, involving the destruction of the fetal skull in order to allow it to pass through the birth canal. This could be by crushing, or by perforation using some kind of scissors (Ryan, 2002:464), or possibly a combination of the two (Churchill, 2003:26).
2   Embryotomy, comprising the destruction and removal of the baby's body, possibly after the fetal skull had been reduced by craniotomy (Ryan, 2002:464). Instruments such as the 'hook' and the 'crochet' would have been used.

As well as destroying the baby, though, these interventions invariably damaged the mother.

The application of obstetric forceps, unlike the 'hook' or the 'crochet', at least carried the *potential* to deliver the baby alive. The risk to the mother of trauma, haemorrhage and infection tends to have been disregarded as does injury to the baby. These forceps were intended to be applied in a situation of a marginally contracted pelvis or in a case of dystocia or uterine inertia.

In cases of contracted pelvis giving rise to cephalo-pelvic disproportion, interventions to enlarge the bony pelvis have, as an alternative, been variably fashionable. These operations vary in their approach, but are named according to the structure being divided to enlarge the pelvis (Churchill, 2003:24).

1   Symphysiotomy is a form of pelviotomy in which the cartilaginous joint in the anterior part of the pelvis is divided (Skippen et al, 2004). The success rate of this intervention was dire as: 'Approximately a third of mothers and two thirds of children died after the operation' (Skippen et al, 2004:59). Although some may still favour this operation and regard it as lifesaving (Bjorklund, 2002: Wykes et al, 2003), women who have experienced it appear to hold a different view (SOS, 2002).
2   Pubiotomy comprises the division of the pubic bones (Comer, 1921).
3   Hebeosteotomy is another form of pelviotomy which involves 'cutting the pubic bone just lateral to the symphysis pubis' (Wenger, 2000:276).

These operations, though, carry serious risks of life-threatening bleeding and laceration of the woman's genital tissues, as well as longer term problems of fistula formation leading to constant urinary incontinence. Additionally, impaired mobility is a long-term problem; if walking is ever to be possible again, a prolonged period of immobility, with the attendant risks of thrombo-embolic disorders, is required.

In the care of women with contracted pelvis, attempts could be made to avoid caesarean by seeking to deliver a baby small enough to pass through the pathologically reduced pelvic diameters. This may have been by attempting to either limit fetal growth by effectively starving the woman or by the premature induction of the labour and delivery (Comer, 1921:314).

Clearly, this litany of potential disasters demonstrates the extreme measures to which the obstetrician would resort in order to avoid the use of caesarean. The reason for this avoidance was indisputably the operation's phenomenally high mortality rates. A major cause of maternal, and possibly fetal, mortality was infection following a prolonged labour. Vaginal examinations and other interventions would introduce pathogens. If a caesarean were to be performed, these organisms would contaminate the abdominal cavity, causing peritonitis followed by paralytic ileus, a form of intestinal obstruction. Caesarean carried a risk of peritonitis even in the absence of prolonged labour, because suturing of the uterus was deemed unnecessary; the logic being that third stage and subsequent contractions would close the wound (de Costa, 2001:98; Hem and Børdahl, 2003). The unsutured uterus, though, would discharge the lochia, rich in potentially infected uterine debris, into the peritoneal cavity. This release of lochia was able to be prevented by the, to modern eyes, rather extreme measures of ligation of the cervix or else by hysterectomy.

The historical rationale for needing to avoid caesarean becomes abundantly clear in the maternal mortality rates associated with this operation. Trolle reports the number of caesareans in Britain from 1737 to 1878 as 131. The maternal mortality rate for caesarean over this 141-year period was 83 per cent (1982:37). Excruciatingly high as this figure may now appear, it compares favourably with caesarean's 100 per cent maternal mortality in Paris over a similar period (Ainsworth, 2003). Clearly, the caesarean operation has changed out of all recognition since obstetricians endeavoured at all costs to avoid surgical intervention. It may be, though, that instead of the situation becoming simpler with the development of different surgical and anaesthetic techniques, it has become more complicated. For this reason, I argue that the benefits of a surgical birth may not be totally unmitigated.

1.3 Changes in caesarean rates

In spite of these dire maternal outcomes, medical practitioners' enthusiasm for this operation and the chances of fetal and maternal survival continued to increase. Jacques René Tenon (1788) provides a baseline for tracing how practice changed. He reports 79 successful caesareans having been undertaken in Europe in the preceding 288 years.

Because of the general British wariness of the operation, the first successful caesarean in England was not performed until 1793. The reason for this caution appears in observations that, while the number of caesareans undertaken in Britain gradually increased in the late eighteenth and early nineteenth centuries, the survival rate (if anything) deteriorated from 29 to 18 per cent (Churchill, 2003). Meanwhile, in continental Europe and North America, the survival rate was both higher and more stable at just below 50 per cent.

Trolle (1982) takes up the story by reporting the caesarean rate in one Danish maternity hospital from 1870 to 1975. Beginning with a caesarean rate of approximately 0.2 per cent and a mortality rate of 100 per cent, by 1975 the caesarean rate had risen to over 17 per cent and the maternal mortality rate had fallen to just below 0.1 per cent.

This general pattern of a reduction in the negative correlation between caesarean rates and maternal mortality is exemplified in the UK Confidential Enquiries (MacFarlane, 2004). This weakening link was effectively dealt the *coup de grâce* by the introduction of regional anaesthesia (Mander, 1993a). It may be that the reduction in the risk of maternal mortality by the easy availability of anaesthesia served to fuel the exponential rise in the caesarean rate of the late twentieth century (Figure 1.1).

This introduction to the crucially important, yet fiendishly complex, matter of caesarean rates is intended to provide simply an overview of the historical and recent developments. More attention is given to caesarean rates in subsequent chapters, such as the incidence of emergency and elective operations (Chapter 3), international comparisons (Chapter 4) and issues associated with a subsequent birth (Chapter 8). Even this simplistic introduction to the caesarean rates, though, does

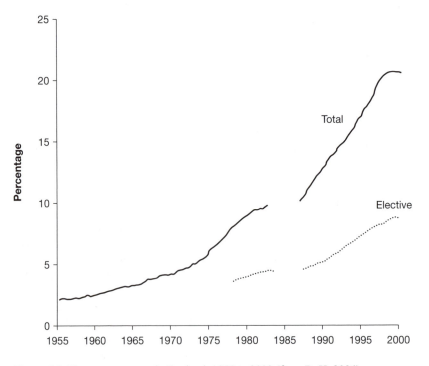

Figure 1.1 The caesarean rate in England, 1955 to 2002 (from DoH, 2004).

serve to provide an indication of just one of the reasons why this intervention is so important. I continue now to introduce some of the reasons why caesarean matters so much to childbearing women, to those who provide maternity care, to policy makers and to human society as a whole.

1.4 The significance of caesarean

The changes in rates, by themselves, clearly indicate why caesarean is such an important topic. In merely numerical terms, caesarean matters because the incidence is increasing despite all efforts to control it; additionally, however, the implications for women, for their babies and their families require attention. To these essential considerations should be added the consequences for both the formal and the informal care providers.

Because of the increasing incidence of caesarean, it may be that this operation is becoming little more than just another kind of birth; this applies to the extent that it may sometimes even be regarded as a 'normal' procedure. The meaning of the term 'normal', as it is widely used in childbearing, is clearly in need of careful attention. This analysis of 'normal' raises questions about the interventions which are frequently, and perhaps even routinely, used in maternity care. Thus, there is a discussion of the meaning of interventions and their place, which leads to an analysis of the ongoing debate on the cascade of intervention.

1.4.1 The woman

The mother has been criticised for being selfish for wanting a caesarean on the grounds of being 'too posh to push'. Paradoxically, she has also been criticised for not wanting a caesarean on the grounds that she is selfishly prioritising her own wishes over her baby's health and welfare. Caesarean may be yet another of those situations where a woman's place is in the wrong. Research, such as that by Weaver (2000), is now beginning to fill the gaps in our understanding of the complexities of the woman's birth decision making. The implications of caesarean for the woman are addressed in detail in Chapters 6 and 7.

1.4.2 The baby

While the assumption is commonly made that being squeezed through the birth canal may not be the best entry into the world, evidence is accumulating which suggests that this assumption is wrong. As well as the longstanding realisation that vaginal birth actually benefits neonatal pulmonary function (Milner et al, 1978), other evidence is being brought to light. These research studies relate to the association of caesarean with neurological problems, allergies and lacerations. Caesarean's implications for the neonate are examined in Chapters 5 and 6.

1.4.3 The midwife

Perhaps unsurprisingly, some midwives question whether the midwife's role may be threatened by the increasing caesarean rates. For this reason, if for no other, caesarean is of immense importance to the midwife. Some midwives are responding assertively to this potential threat by focusing on their role in facilitating 'normality' in childbearing (see section 1.4.8). Other midwives are endeavouring to ground their approach to care more firmly in the multidisciplinary team (Warwick, 2001). So, rather than the midwife retreating to her own specialised area of expertise in 'normal' childbearing, she is being urged to build bridges with other disciplines, supposedly in the interests of the childbearing family. In Chapter 7, I consider the issues which caesarean raises for the midwife.

1.4.4 The obstetrician

The medical view of caesarean may be interpreted as paradoxical to the point of being schizoid. While some obstetricians argue fervently for the need to reduce the number of caesareans, others regard this development as their contribution to evolution (see Chapter 9). The 'research' by Al-Mufti and colleagues, though, casts doubt on any medical adherence to the reduction of caesarean rates (1997). This research, which is examined more fully in Chapter 8, clearly demonstrates the dependence of obstetricians on caesarean. This dependence is shown to prevail not only in the professional arena but, more importantly, in their personal and domestic lives. I address the implications of caesarean for the medical profession in Chapters 8 and 9.

1.4.5 The manager/policy-maker

For those who plan and manage health systems and maternity services the increasing number of caesareans may not be an unmixed blessing. On the one hand, this intervention permits the efficient planning of services and the most effective use of limited resources. On the other hand, because econometric analyses of the financial costs of caesarean are ambiguous, this operation's more frequent use may be aggravating the spiralling health care costs. Even for those analysts, though, who argue the cost-effectiveness of caesarean, future costs of subsequent births by caesarean and their complications are unlikely to be taken into account. In Chapters 2 and 3 I consider the significance of caesarean for policy makers and managers.

1.4.6 Politics

The inherently political nature of reproduction and childbearing is only now beginning to gain the acceptance and attention which it deserves (Clement, 1995:xix). The political manoeuvring around childbearing features the changing balance of power between the various actors. These include between the woman and the care providers, between the different disciplines in attendance, between female participants and their male counterparts and between those involved whose focus is the baby and those who prioritise the woman's experience. I attempt to recognise the political implications of caesarean throughout this book.

1.4.7 General population

That humans have been giving birth vaginally since they first came into being does not need to be stated. While it is necessary to admit that spontaneous birth may not invariably function perfectly, it carries the advantage that it is something that the woman does, rather than having it done to her. Such a profound change in an activity as fundamentally human as childbirth can only have momentous consequences, although what those consequences are is not yet clear. I adopt a philosophical stance in Chapter 8 to contemplate the really long-term picture of these developments.

Since our Victorian great-grandparents could only bring themselves to refer to pregnancy as 'an interesting condition', attitudes have changed markedly. While previously the ultimate unmentionables, sex and childbearing have become a major focus of media attention and death has now taken their place as taboo (Gorer, 1965). The popular media are perceived as a major provider of information about matters such as caesarean (Beech, 2000b). Their commercial and, hence, sensationalist orientation allows limited opportunities for serious analysis of the issues. Any in-depth consideration of these crucial issues is likely to be relegated to broadsheets and late night slots. Beech argues that even female journalists are likely to be either ignorant, prejudiced or both. Such prejudices may be founded on unfortunate personal experience, but they still preclude any degree of objectivity. Midwives' limited media-literacy is a source of regret (Warwick, 2001); thus, Victoria Beckham's caesarean attracts many more column inches than Cherie Blair's normal birth.

1.4.8 'Normal' childbearing

As mentioned above (see section 1.4.3), caesarean in particular and medicalisation in general may be perceived by some midwives as a threat to their role. One response to this has been an increased emphasis on the role carved out for midwives as being to focus solely on 'normal' childbearing. Whether this strategy is likely to be successful depends very much on the meaning which is ascribed to 'normal'. Like a number of words, this is one which can be interpreted in many ways and which may vary according to the values of the person using it. It may be that 'normal' is one of those Alice in Wonderland words: 'When I say a word, it means what I want it to mean, nothing more and nothing less' (Carroll, 2000: 221).

In her concept analysis of 'normal labour', Gould (2000) sought to clarify this Wonderland word and identified five distinct ways in which the term could be used.

- Normality has been defined in statistical terms to indicate the most frequently occurring, that is the median, or the average or mean. Unfortunately, these definitions say little about the woman's experience or the midwife's contribution and more about the environment of routinisation in which the birth happens.
- 'Upright' is another interpretation of normal, which Gould links to the woman's posture in physiological labour.
- 'Healthy' is also offered by Gould as a synonym for normal. This term, however, may be unhelpful because every birth should be maintained within the bounds of good health, but the means by which this is achieved may be anything but physiological.
- For some women 'normal' may have become an ideal for which to strive. Clearly, the subjectivity of this meaning renders it useless without probing.
- Normal meaning 'not pathological', I suggest, carries an aura of objectivity, but this may be spurious because the pathology is subject to diagnosis and interpretation.
- 'Natural' may be the least unsatisfactory meaning of normal in Gould's classification. Unfortunately, though, for those of us with long memories, the equation of normal with natural is rendered difficult by its association with American 'natural childbirth'. This referred to any vaginal birth which fell short of the full panoply of interventions, including general anaesthesia, routine episiotomy and prophylactic forceps.

I would like to offer a different meaning of normal which, if not helpful, at least provides food for thought. In order to avoid the confusion between 'what is common and what is normal', 'intervention-free' may appear to be a hopeful interpretation (Beech, 2002b:1). It is obvious that operative and instrumental birth are not included.

With the redefinition of 'normal' as 'intervention-free', the questions soon start to emerge. Particularly difficult is the role of episiotomy or third stage oxytocic drugs in normal childbearing. Thus, it becomes necessary to address an even more challenging question concerning what constitutes an intervention? It may be argued that any external factor which carries the potential to influence the progress of the labour should be included in this category. I venture to suggest, therefore, that even the presence of an attendant, such as a midwife, or the move into a different environment, such as a maternity unit, constitute interventions.

1.4.9 Cascade of intervention

The use of a variety of interventive techniques has led to the identification of the 'cascade of intervention' by some observers of current obstetric practice (Varney Burst, 1983; Kitzinger, 1998). The existence of the cascade has been supported by studies in the UK and in Scandinavia. This phenomenon is associated with an intervention, such as the partograph, altering the progress of labour from a physiological route. To resolve these alterations pharmacological interventions are introduced to augment labour and/or control pain. Oxytocic drugs to augment labour are associated with fetal hypoxia, identified as fetal distress, for which interventions to expedite the birth, such as assistance with obstetric forceps or even caesarean section, may be deemed necessary. Thus, an iatrogenic progression may manifest itself. This begins with interventions which, *per se*, are relatively benign, but which may lead inexorably to the ultimate 'rescue operation' which is the focus of this book.

This cascade is obviously the subject of some controversy. The authoritative work of Cheyne and her colleagues (2003) suggests that one intervention, the routine 'admission strip', has been found 'not guilty' of initiating the cascade. These researchers argue that, in spite of this verdict, the effect of the culture of the labour ward setting merits research attention. Cheyne and her colleagues clearly believe that the cascade of intervention is alive and well, even though their research on the admission strip did not locate it.

1.5 Conclusion

In this introductory chapter, I have taken the opportunity to outline some of the crucial caesarean-related issues, some of which will re-emerge later in this book. Of particular interest, though, is the paradox which arises out of the examination of the history of the caesarean. This shows that it is a surgical operation which seems likely to have begun as little more than a way of avoiding a coffin birth, which was perceived as being disagreeable to the point of disaster. Through etymological, hagiographical and fashionable influences, this operation has become imbued with an aura of supernatural power, as found in the myths of Julius Caesar, Scipio and Macduff. This may be attributable to it sharing a name with one of those superheroes. As mentioned already the German language name for the oper-ation, '*der Kaiserschnitt*', also endorses the operation's imperial credentials.

The importance of the name in increasing the acceptability and incidence of this operation is difficult to assess, but I would argue that the name may have done the operation no harm at all in terms of its widespread acceptance. The link with those of noble birth, of greatness, even if it was mythological, and superhuman powers may have been persuasive that it was not just a 'rescue operation'. This is evident in Trolle's observation that caesarean has become regarded as 'the godly way to enter the world' (1982:9).

2 What are the questions and who's using the answers? Research into caesarean

Does research really matter in areas as fundamentally important as the survival of a newborn baby? If a woman has been in labour for twenty hours, does research help with the decision about whether a caesarean should be undertaken? Some would say that any intervention which has the potential to save the life of a newborn must, by definition, be justified. Such arguments, well intentioned though they are, neglect the nuances of judgement, as well as the delicate balance between risks and benefits for both the mother and the baby. Thus, rather than being an irrelevance, I would suggest that research becomes even more significant; this significance is only enhanced by the possibility that interventions such as caesarean may be misused.

In order to look at the role of research *vis à vis* caesarean, I offer, first, a 'health warning' about the relevance and use of research. Next I examine the main research approaches and then the implementation or non-implementation of this research. This leads on to a brief consideration of research ethics. Then, in order to establish the applicability of the research to which I refer, I scrutinise the possibility of different origins of the research and any implications which these various origins may carry. Next I consider, by way of illustration, two aspects of caesarean which have been subjected to research, one of which demonstrates admirably many of the crucial issues. On the basis of my consideration of these two aspects, I indicate some areas which are still in need of research attention.

2.1 A 'health warning'

In contemplating the research on caesarean, it is crucial to bear in mind the sources of that research. By this, I mean that much of the research and other material have originated in countries and from disciplines which may have their own cultures and their own agenda. It is possible that these agendas may be different from those of the childbearing woman and other users of the research findings. A particularly notable or notorious example may be found in the USA. There is a serious obsession there about the escalating costs of health care (Harer, 2002). This obsession and these costs are being aggravated by the relatively frequent use of caesarean there (see Chapter 3). These factors, if linked with the different funding of the health system, lead to agendas which may differ from those of the childbearing woman and from other countries. Thus, in interpreting the research literature, it is necessary to remember the different cultures, disciplines and health care systems in the countries from which much of the research and other literature originate. It may be helpful to question the relevance of such research to the woman and to her health care providers in their own environment.

2.2 Randomised Controlled Trials and Evidence-Based Practice

It was as far away and long ago as Vienna in 1847 that Ignaz Semmelweis undertook his hugely important controlled trial to demonstrate the cause of puerperal sepsis (Ayliffe and English, 2003:61). In spite of Semmelweis's pioneering work, in the field of health care generally, the value of the randomised controlled trial (RCT) only started to be widely recognised towards the end of the twentieth century. This recognition arose out of concerns about the questionable benefits of certain forms of treatment, as well as the high costs of health care. The RCT has come to be widely regarded as a major research tool for finding out what interventions are safe, as well as both effective and efficient. This high regard is exemplified in the observation by Enkin and his colleagues, who maintain that the logic underpinning the RCT, if implemented conscientiously, makes this research design 'the gold standard for comparing alternative forms of care' (1995:70). Thus, the RCT is able to provide accurate information or 'evidence' to assist decisions about the form of care to be offered in a clinical setting. To assist the clinician in this way, the Cochrane Library (2005) provides an impressive list of 33 caesarean-related systematic reviews of RCTs. It is not impossible that some of this research was stimulated by longstanding criticisms of obstetrics' pathetic research foundation, such as the comments by Cochrane in 1972. His scathing critique of the practice of obstetricians has, at least, increased the likelihood of a firm foundation for future evidence-based practice (EBP).

Although the rhetoric of RCTs and EBP has been widely espoused, dissenting voices have been raised to question the relevance of this dogma to childbearing and to midwifery. This dissent has grown out of the realisation that research evidence alone is not an adequate basis for the care of the childbearing woman. As has been suggested in a midwifery context, the evidence needs to be 'moderated by the midwife's occupational experience, personal experience of childbearing and intuitive knowledge' (Mander, 2006a). A crucial adjunct to these moderating factors is, of course, the woman's own personal knowledge and experience.

These more womanly forms of knowledge are essential to midwifery care, in view of the fundamental humanity of childbearing. Due to this, the relevance of RCTs and other forms of quantitative research has been criticised on the grounds of their 'reductionist' approach. This is because, in order to make sense of the respondents' behaviour or responses, the researcher may need to simplify or 'reduce' the phenomena to their most basic component parts. This reductionism may be regarded as a strength, in that it serves to highlight and clarify important issues. There is, however, a risk that such a reductionist approach to an area as human and complex as childbearing may ignore some vital aspect. This may be due to the researcher being unaware of the existence of this aspect or, possibly, because it is too complex, or otherwise challenging, to be addressed (Mander, 1999).

These concerns about the mismatch between the care of the childbearing woman and the RCT/EBP dogma are reflected in others' writing (Jowitt, 2001). Additionally, Jowitt demonstrates the disparity between the 'hands off' (2001:9) nature of midwifery, and the centrality of interventions and their testing in RCTs. That midwifery is fundamentally non-interventive is summarised in the familiar translation of 'midwife' as being 'with woman'. Jowitt builds on the perceptive ideas of Banks (2001), who effectively 're-frames' the debate in terms of research evidence being a medical device, which is alien to the midwifery role. Banks argues that the essential and uniquely individual nature of childbearing conflicts with the large randomised samples required by RCTs and EBP. Presenting views that to some may appear heretical, Banks argues that the midwife should be listening to the individual woman, rather than endeavouring to manoeuvre her midwifery practice to conform to the EBP straitjacket.

The writings of Jowitt (2001) and of Banks (2001) demonstrate some of the misgivings held by midwives about the ways in which RCTs are used in maternity care. Their concerns resonate with the work of Wiggins and Newburn (2004) who, in the context of providing evidence-based information, collected women's views about EBP. These researchers found that women were suitably wary of research evidence, preferring to think in terms of concrete situations, real staff and their own preferences. As well as these background concerns, their informants also wished to be told:

- the kinds of research methods used
- who carried out the research
- the number of women involved
- when the research was carried out (2004:157).

It may be because of concerns like these that, as early as 1991, the gap between the research evidence and its implementation started to become apparent (Funk et al, 1991). Thus, to paraphrase Florence Nightingale, it was realised that research evidence is not 'self-executive' (1863). The existence of this gap has continued to be problematical, and whether it is bridgeable is yet to be seen. The factors which engender this gap and which act as impediments to evidence-based practice (EBP) have been revisited on a regular basis since 1991. The findings have usually been similar to those of McKenna and colleagues (2004), who showed that the culture of clinical practice needs to change if evidence-based practice is to become a reality. On the basis of this discussion of the place of EBP in maternity care, it is necessary to conclude that it is 'a good thing'. Like many good things, though, the reality may fall short of the rhetoric. This shortfall applies particularly in terms of EBP dogma being demanded of occupational groups, such as midwives, who have other appropriate sources of knowledge; particularly galling is the tendency of these demands to be made by other occupational groups whose EBP credentials are far from complete.

2.3 Research ethics and caesarean

The limited implementation of research inevitably raises questions about the morality of undertaking research which is not actually put into operation. It may be that not using research is as unethical as the widespread practice of undertaking research which is never disseminated (Mander, 1996a). I venture to suggest that the non-dissemination or non-implementation of a study renders that research unethical, on the grounds of the misuse of the resources devoted to the research. Additionally, the involvement of the subjects may constitute a form of abuse, because of the inconvenience, if not the potential for harm, to which they have been exposed.

In her analysis of the ethics of midwifery research, Hicks (2004) focuses on the RCT to demonstrate how some research may offend against the basic ethical principles of research. She maintains that the RCT flouts the ethical principles of beneficence, non-maleficence, fidelity and justice. This disregard will be further compounded by any pre-existing suspicion that either the intervention or the standard treatment is 'superior' (2004:274). She goes on to demonstrate that these criticisms are not mere academic pedantry. They are exacerbated by the fact that RCT findings, like other data, are vulnerable to deliberate distortion in the interests, as Hicks puts it, of 'academic and professional promotion' (2004:275).

The concept and practice of randomisation, which are fundamental aspects of the RCT, present many difficulties to those who are not familiar with them (Robinson, 2005). Some people approached to participate in an RCT will assume that the 'new' treatment is inevitably preferable to the standard treatment. Other potential participants may assume that randomisation is a method of allocating scarce resources, like the all too familiar 'postcode lottery'. For some, there may be difficulty believing that a medical intervention might be being employed if it is anything other than entirely safe and effective. Similarly, research by Robinson and colleagues (2004) found that health care consumers could not believe that a clinician might be genuinely uncertain about the relative harms and benefits of two different treatments. To the majority of this sample of members of the public, the concept of randomisation for treatment was abhorrent. These researchers conclude that the RCT may carry a number of ethical problems; not least among these is the difficulty which the potential participants experience in understanding what is involved.

Research into caesarean is no different from any other area, in that it raises a multiplicity of ethical issues. One of these issues, identified by Robertson (2003), relates to the questionable ethical status of a proposed RCT to evaluate the benefits and hazards of caesarean for healthy first time mothers. She questions the rationale for undertaking such an RCT, blaming private health care provided by male obstetricians in wealthy western states. The argument which emerges is a plea for more resources to be channelled into ensuring uncomplicated births attended by midwives.

Further ethical concerns are raised by an intended systematic review of 'secondary caesarean' versus vaginal birth after caesarean or VBAC (see Chapter 8)

(Dodd et al, 2004). My MEDLINE (1966–2006) search, though, suggests that these reviewers are likely to encounter difficulty. Using the search terms 'VBAC' or 'Vaginal birth after caesarean' and 'Trial of labour' or 'Trial of Labor', my search produced 739 hits. However, when 'RCT' was added to each of these terms, there were no hits whatsoever. Thus, using an authoritative database, I have been unable to identify any RCTs focusing on vaginal birth after a caesarean.

It is not hard to imagine why this should be. In order to undertake such an RCT, it would be necessary to recruit a suitable sample of women. This would involve pregnant women being given complete information about the issues, including the possible risks of each type of birth. On the basis of this information, each woman would be asked to consent to being randomised into one mode of birth group or the other; that is elective repeat caesarean or trial of labour with a view to VBAC. It is likely that, even if such a study were to be given ethical and managerial approval, women would have serious misgivings about being randomised. This lack of relevant RCTs is, I suggest, likely to persist in spite of the optimism of Dodd and her colleagues.

An ethical problem which may occur in the context of research into, particularly emergency, caesarean relates to the meaning of consent. While all researchers pay lip service to the ideal of informed consent, the reality may differ. This is because of the consent being given 'under difficult conditions' (Robinson, 2005:4), when the woman may feel pressured into making a decision without the usual 'thinking time':

> women are often asked to consent to take part in research while they are actually in labour. At such a time women will usually be unable to give their full attention to the details of the research project. They are likely to be coping with painful contractions, they may have been given drugs and they may be anxious about possible complications.
>
> (AIMS/NCT, 1997:2)

Whether the woman is fit to take in information and to give consent to being involved in research is questionable, so any consent which she gives may be invalid. The pressure which the woman may feel not to antagonise her care providers by not agreeing to their invitation may further invalidate her consent.

The AIMS/NCT Charter emphasises the need for the woman to be given information well ahead of her being asked to consent to participate; hence the 'thinking time' mentioned already. This would mean information being given during pregnancy, in appropriate language and format and with opportunities for questions or discussion. Of particular importance is the woman's right to either see the results or, at least, to be told how to access the results. This Charter, unlike some agencies, attaches equal importance to both experimental and 'social science' research, considering that both comprise an intervention which may have long-term consequences for the mother and baby. AIMS/NCT concludes that childbearing research should involve women and consumer representatives at an early stage in the planning of any research project, thus: 'Research should be undertaken with women, not on women' (1997:5).

Other ethical issues relating to caesarean research, as well as some examples of the issues mentioned already, emerge out of the 'case study' of the Term Breech Trial (see section 2.5.2 below).

2.4 The origins of caesarean research

In reading any research report, it is advisable to scrutinise carefully the authors' details, including gender, occupations and affiliations. This investment of time provides a wealth of background information which is likely to facilitate understanding and interpretation of the research and its conclusions. While this scrutiny may be just for academic purposes, it is a necessary precursor to decisions about the use or implementation of research.

2.4.1 The geographical location

The location of the research, which may be ascertained from the authors' affiliations, is likely to hint at the relevance of the research to one's own health care environment.

One example may be found in the research by Béhague and colleagues (2002) who report that in Brazil, 55 per cent of moderately affluent women give birth by caesarean. This figure serves to conceal a caesarean rate of '80% to 90%' in some private hospitals (Béhague et al, 2002:943). These researchers found that Brazilian women have complex reasons for seeking to undergo this operation. For these reasons, the Brazilian woman is likely to use a number of manoeuvres in order to avoid giving birth vaginally. The underlying rationale, though, is the woman's determination to avoid the abysmally poor care provided for women experiencing an uncomplicated birth. Thus, undergoing this major surgery is the only way for the Brazilian woman to obtain an acceptable standard of care. It is apparent that these women do not necessarily regard caesarean as a desirable way to give birth, but it is the least bad of the options available. Unfortunately, a brief glance at the title of Béhague and colleagues' paper 'Consumer demand for caesarean sections in Brazil: informed decision making, patient choice, or social inequality?' may be misleading. Cursory attention to this title might lead the average reader of the *British Medical Journal* to assume that women in Brazil, as some would like to believe is the case in the northern hemisphere, are demanding caesareans. Thus, the context of the research, in this case the appalling care for Brazilian women in 'normal labour', becomes crucial to our understanding of the research findings.

2.4.2 The researchers' discipline

In reading any research report, it is always helpful to understand from where the researchers are coming. This applies not only in terms of the geographical origins mentioned already, but also in relation to their disciplinary background. It is hardly surprising that researchers may, according to their disciplines, have differing views and agendas. While I am in no way suggesting that the findings or the data are likely to be affected by the researchers' professional origins, it is not impossible that the research questions and the research approaches will be thus influenced.

An important example was the ground-breaking work by Hillan (1991a,b; 1992a,b,c; 1995). As an exemplary midwife researcher, Hillan's research illuminated many important aspects of the sequelae of the caesarean operation. These included crucial areas, such as the woman's limited understanding of the reasons for the caesarean being performed. Hillan also brought to light the short-term and the long-term health problems which follow after caesarean (see Chapters 6 and 7). While these problems did not affect the woman's or the baby's survival, they did affect how the woman was able to adjust to motherhood following the caesarean. As a midwife, Hillan could quite appropriately have interviewed a sample of women, but she chose not to do this. She collected her data by sending a postal questionnaire to 588 women three months after they had had a caesarean. The data were analysed quantitatively to provide an overall picture of women's poor health after the operation. Whether Hillan's choice of research approach was influenced by her being based in a Department of Nursing Studies which was housed in a Faculty of Medicine is difficult to assess. But the structured postal questionnaire as a research tool is notorious for the superficial nature of the data collected; this is due largely to the respondent's inability to clarify the questions (Rees, 1997). Thus, it may be argued that Hillan's findings would have been more sensitive had she used a more woman-friendly, and less medically determined method of data collection.

In the same way, consideration needs to be given to the research undertaken by Crowther's medical team in Adelaide, Australia. This research team has already been mentioned in the discussion of Dodd et al's questionably ethical plans to research VBAC (please see section 2.3 above). Whether Dodd's uncertain ethical position reflects a more general obstetric view of research ethics would be unclear. In this medical setting, though, the RCT appears to be the research method of choice.

The qualitative research project by Clement, on the other hand, provides a greater depth of understanding of the woman's experience. It may be that this depth befits Clement's disciplinary background as a psychologist. Her qualitative approach to her study resulted in a surprisingly large number of informants, 'two hundred women' (1995:xviii) in all. The questionnaires which the women completed sought their experiences and feelings and gave the women apparently infinite space to reply. The result was that some of the women wrote more than a dozen pages on their feelings about their experiences. In this way, Clement's profound findings do justice to the magnitude of the experiences which the women recount. Unfortunately, her account of the research is less rigorous, with the method and the analysis of the data being given scant consideration.

2.4.3 The researcher's personal experience

An area which attracts considerable interest among informants and respondents is the researcher's reason for undertaking a particular project. Particularly important is whether and how it relates to the researcher's personal experience. This personal involvement has been crucial to a number of projects which I have undertaken (Mander, 1995a; 2001b).

It may be that this level of personal interest is necessary to motivate the researcher during the difficult times when the research is not progressing according to the plan. Alternatively, the researcher may be seeking, through the research, to exorcise her own 'ghosts'; in this way the researcher may be endeavouring to use the research as a form of therapy. This was the background to a research project looking at caesarean by an American campaigning group:

> Young, who still experiences pain three years later, immersed herself in researching caesarean births as part of her healing process. Because of her background in zoology and her experience in proving theories through research, she took an evidence-based approach.
>
> (ICAN, 2004)

The question which remains, though, is whether and to what extent personal experience may have an effect on the research itself. Personal experience of childbearing is widely held to be crucially important to the practice of a midwife (Mander, 1996b). The value of such experience, though, is contested by midwives who have not borne children. Could it be that the importance of childbearing experience to the researcher is similarly contentious? For Sarah Clement her experience of giving birth by caesarean appears to have been fundamental to her supremely insightful caesarean research. As well as her many other attributes Clement describes herself as a 'caesarean mother' (1995). While she does not provide details about the nature of her caesarean experience, she does thank her son, whose birth inspired her to undertake the research.

In the case of Clement, her personal experience of caesarean clearly helps her to identify with other mothers who have had similar experiences. It may be difficult to imagine that such experience may have any disadvantages. While personal bias and lack of objectivity are not apparent in this example, it is possible to imagine that in some circumstances they might feature. It is only possible to surmise whether these uncertainties also apply to the researcher's occupational experience. For example, it may be that certain occupational groups are more likely, or possibly less likely, to access an accurate impression of the experience of undergoing a caesarean. To continue the reference to Clement's research, her background as a psychologist may have facilitated her empathetic insights into the caesarean experience.

2.4.4 The timing of the data collection

In research in the maternity field the where and when of the data collection are both interdependent and likely to influence the data. This is because most women give birth in a maternity unit. If the woman is questioned while in the maternity unit, the institutional environment is likely, to say the least, to affect the woman's answers to any questions about events which may have happened there. Thus, it is necessary to look carefully at any study which includes data which were collected during the woman's stay in the maternity unit.

Further, there is some uncertainty about the point of time at which a researcher may be confident that she is tapping in to the woman's genuine and stable feelings about her childbirth experience. Oakley (1993) was confident at six weeks that she was able to access the woman's considered views about the control of her labour pain. On the other hand, Waldenström found that more time needed to elapse before women were able to express their considered views (2004). Waldenström surmises that the initial euphoria, that labour is completed and the baby is healthy, may 'colour' the woman's earlier reactions (2004:102). She goes on to suggest that it takes more time for the woman to be able to face the reality of the less positive aspects of the labour and birth. Such aspects may include the duration of labour, unwelcome medical procedures and unsatisfactory interpersonal relationships. Additionally, there are other aspects of motherhood which may cause the woman to take a more critical view of her experience; these include factors relating to the baby or to her psychosocial environment.

For these all of these reasons, caesarean-related research needs to be scrutinised carefully and critically if the reader is to identify material which may be relevant to her own situation.

2.5 Research topics

As well as the origins of the caesarean research providing a wealth of information to those interested in it, the actual areas which have been addressed by research also provide an indication of what is considered to be important. This assumption of importance derives from any published research having started as a question in the mind of the researcher; it must have mattered sufficiently for the researcher to take the project forward. Additionally, the topic must have been accepted as important enough to be given research ethical approval and management approval. Similarly, the significance of the topic must also have been recognised by a funding body for it to have been completed and published.

In order to provide a broad picture of the aspects of caesarean which have attracted research attention, I have used the Cochrane Library database. After this I focus down on two areas which have attracted the interest of researchers and raise some important issues.

The Cochrane Library database provides a list of the topics which have been or are intended to be subjected to systematic review. This should provide at least an impression of the relative importance attached to the various topics. By entering the word 'caesarean' as the title search term, 32 Cochrane reviews were identified, addressing a range of topics (see Table 2.1).

The largest proportion (40.6 per cent) of reviews addressed techniques used at the time of the operation. These included the site of the surgical incision into the woman's abdomen, the materials used to close the skin wound, the position of the woman during surgery and the mode of delivery of the placenta. This large

Table 2.1 Areas addressed in caesarean-related Cochrane reviews

Topic of review	Number	%
Technique at operation	13	40.6
Anaesthesia/analgesia	5	15.6
Indications	4	12.5
Postnatal/postoperative	4	12.5
Decision	4	12.5
Information to mother	1	3.1
Reducing unnecessary	1	3.1
Total	**32**	**100**

proportion suggests that ideas about the actual technique for the operation are still being investigated with a view to undergoing change and possibly improvement.

The second largest group of reviews related to the anaesthesia used during the operation, which is closely linked with the method of pain control afterwards. These issues were the focus of 15.6 per cent of the reviews and they included techniques to prevent hypotension as a complication of spinal anaesthesia and the use of rectal analgesia for the early postoperative period.

Matters relating to the caesarean decision, to the postoperative period, and to the medical indications for caesarean each comprised 12.5 per cent of the reviews.

The two topics which were addressed least frequently were those which addressed most directly the concerns of the mother. The focus of one of these was 'Information for pregnant women about caesarean birth' (Horey et al, 2004) and the other was 'Non-clinical interventions for reducing unnecessary caesarean section' (Khunpradit et al, 2005). The first of these 'woman-centred' reviews was a full review examining the findings of two RCTs. The second, though, was just a protocol. This means that the systematic review has not yet been completed, so only the objectives are able to be provided and that no abstract or data are yet available.

On the basis of this, admittedly cursory, examination of the topics addressed by one research database, what is clearly apparent is the limited research attention given to those matters which are of direct concern to the woman. The technical issues attract far more research interest than the human, woman-related topics. For this reason, it may be necessary to consider the extent to which those who perform the caesarean are concerned about the woman experiencing this operation as opposed to the operation as an end in itself.

2.5.1 Researching caesarean – information giving

It is clear that, according to the Cochrane Library, a major health research database, the woman's view of caesarean tends to be neglected. It may be helpful at this point to examine this situation in more detail. The woman's experience of caesarean comprises a multiplicity of different aspects. To further complicate matters, depending on where they are coming from, women may interpret the same phenomenon in different ways. For this reason, I seek to explore here research relating to one crucial aspect of the woman's experience. This aspect is information giving.

It probably does not need to be said that information is fundamental to the decision making on which the woman's control over her childbirth experience is founded (please see Chapter 5). The degree of the woman's control is closely associated with the balance of power that exists between her and her attendants. Thus, because health care providers may assume that they are also the major information providers, information giving and power are inextricably interrelated.

That health care providers may have their own agendas was demonstrated in an authoritative research project on the use of evidence-based leaflets to provide information (Stapleton, 2004). These professional agendas may relate to factors as varied as personal childbearing experience, knowledge of research or fear of litigation. The availability of relevant, research-based information may also be included as one of these agendas. The deficiencies of the evidence base, in the specific context of psychological issues associated with caesarean, have been outlined by Clement (2001:110). She shows how the research evidence tends to focus narrowly on a small number of easily researched topics. Even in these well-researched areas, though, the quality of the research does not allow it to be considered as 'strong evidence'. This is because the samples tend to be small and the research design retrospective. The researchers may group women together in different ways, such as by parity or by childbearing experience. The plethora of different instruments and data collection techniques further limits the comparison of findings or the systematic review of studies. As mentioned above (see section 2.4.1) the cultural milieu also affects findings, so multicentre studies may be problematical. The challenge which remains relates to the difficulty of providing sound evidence-based information on topics where that evidence base is still woefully inadequate.

Even in subjects where evidence has been developed, limitations to information giving still persist. As emerged in the study by Stapleton and her colleagues, women sought more than the bare abstract facts in order to make decisions. As one medical practitioner observed:

> Giving them a choice is not enough. They need to know the reality behind it [vaginal breech birth] . . . about the head getting stuck definitely. You can give them scare stories but you don't even have to do that. You just have to mention a complication. Something like the baby might die . . .
>
> (Stapleton et al, 2002:642)

These researchers conclude that just giving information to childbearing women is far from adequate. Stapleton and her colleagues became acutely aware of the effects of the culture of the health care system in which maternity care is provided – with particular recognition of its hierarchical nature. On the basis of their awareness of the crucial role of culture, they conclude that information giving needs to be part of a coherent strategic policy. In this way, the problems of an imbalance of power in health care in general and in maternity in particular may yet be resolved. It may be, however, that an evolutionary approach will not be sufficient to remedy these systematic problems and something more innovatory is required.

2.5.2 Researching caesarean: the Term Breech Trial (TBT)

The baby is said to be particularly vulnerable to perinatal damage if born presenting by the breech (Penn and Ghaem-Maghami, 2001). A large multicentre RCT was planned to resolve, once and for all, any uncertainties about the preferred mode of birth in the event of a breech presentation. A Canada-based study sought the relative benefits of planned caesarean compared with planned vaginal breech birth (Hannah et al, 2000). By focusing on the outcomes, the researchers reached the unequivocal conclusion that the policy of planned caesarean is better for the baby in terms of lowered mortality and morbidity. These findings of this RCT are probably unsurprising in view of the research approach. Equally unsurprisingly, the findings were warmly welcomed and implemented speedily and enthusiastically. Since the publication of the findings, however, there has been a welter of acrimonious criticism, which has culminated in a demand for the researchers to 'withdraw the conclusion of their TBT' (Glezerman, 2006:24). The implementation and findings of this trial impact not only on the childbearing woman, her baby and the practitioners attending them, but also on researchers in general and people possibly affected by caesarean. For these reasons, this trial merits careful attention.

The *numbers* in the Term Breech Trial are important, mainly because, in the context of an RCT, size does matter. To reach statistical significance, the required sample size was calculated to be 2,800 women with a breech presentation. Unusually, however, the trial was called to a halt before that figure was reached, supposedly on the grounds of the results being overwhelmingly in favour of planned caesarean. In 26 countries, a total of 2,088 women had been recruited in 121 centres (Hannah et al, 2000). The reason given for stopping the study, though, is slightly bizarre in view of the difficulty encountered in recruiting and retaining a suitable sample, particularly of women having a planned vaginal breech birth. The TBT website shows the manoeuvres necessary to reach even the 2,088 women recruited (TBT, 2004); tactics included plaudits and coffee mugs in recognition of successful recruitment. The numbers problem may be at the root of many of the issues which have resulted in criticisms being heaped on this project. Numbers also explain some of the weaknesses or limitations inherent in the TBT. The participants, however, were said to need to be recruited and retained 'at any cost' (Glezerman, 2006:24); as a result, some aspects of the study fall seriously short of accepted and acceptable standards of research behaviour.

There are a number of *methodological* limitations in the Term Breech Trial which serve to further reduce its value. One of these also relates to its size. The researchers had no choice but to embark on a massive multicentre trial because a number of previous RCTs had been unable to address certain crucial issues. This inability was due to the earlier RCTs having been too small to show clinically significant differences between the caesarean and the vaginal birth groups (Kotaska,

2004:1040). Some of the problems relate to the statistical technique known as 'intention to treat analysis' (ITT), which was used in the Term Breech Trial. This technique is usually regarded as 'conservative' because it tends to underestimate differences between the groups. Significantly in this context it carries the advantage that, irrespective of any untoward events, the participants stay not only in the groups to which they were randomised, but also in the study. In his critique, Glezerman (2006:23) examines the relevance of the intention to treat analysis and finds it wanting. His criticism is that ITT is most appropriate to assess treatment policies, as opposed to the outcomes in terms of clients who did or did not receive the planned intervention.

The problem of reaching and maintaining the size of the sample is likely to have influenced *recruitment* practices. This is particularly applicable to the standard of care provided in some of the centres. Certain quite basic criteria were used to classify approximately one third of the centres as providing a 'high standard of care'. These criteria included, for example, the availability of someone to give the newborn baby oxygen by means of a bag and mask; a technique which is certainly not rocket science. It is necessary to question the usefulness of data collected in institutions where even interventions as basic as this are not available. Additionally, many centres did not have regular access to equipment for ultrasound investigations, which may be helpful in confirming the diagnosis of breech presentation. Glezerman goes on to argue that data from centres with such low standards are 'hardly acceptable' and 'not applicable' (2006:21). This criticism is endorsed by the fact that antenatal pelvimetry, another sensible precaution, was also lacking in many of the centres (Uotila et al, 2005).

The lack of access to diagnostic ultrasound in some of the institutions may be the reason for the inclusion in the sample of some women and babies who were outwith the criteria for entry, which stated:

> a singleton live fetus . . . Women were excluded if . . . 4000 g or more . . . a fetal anomaly or a condition that might cause a mechanical problem at the delivery . . .
>
> (Hannah et al, 2000:1375–6)

That these criteria were not applied is evident from the eventual sample, which actually included two sets of twins, one anencephalic fetus, two babies who were stillborn and a baby with a ruptured myelomeningocoele. Thus, questions arise about the extent to which the recruiters were able or prepared to adhere to the entry/exclusion criteria (Glezerman, 2006). Or is it possible that the incentives being offered could not be refused? Perhaps it is understandable that a small number of unfortunate women might inadvertently be recruited. That they and their babies were not excused from the study when the situation was identified is more difficult to understand; until, of course, one recalls the stringent application of the 'intention to treat' dogma.

Thus, it is becoming apparent that the allegedly poorer outcomes for the babies born vaginally may have been due to factors other than the mode of birth. One of these factors may have been the size of the baby, which quite appropriately was set at an upper limit of four kilos. It may be assumed that, as the planned caesarean was recommended to be scheduled for 38 or more weeks, the randomisation should have happened by that date. For women who were randomised to the vaginal birth group, though, the baby could easily continue growing and the skull bones hardening by ossification for a further four weeks. So, although estimated to be less than four kilos at entry to the trial, at birth the baby could be considerably more than that; then the risks to the baby and the mother would be correspondingly greater.

Even though it was clearly crucial that the sample should be large enough to ensure statistical significance, the heterogeneity of this large sample proved unwieldy. Uotila and colleagues argue that the ability to maintain both the quality and the consistency of the *data* over such a variable research site, as well as over the three-year time period, must be 'questionable' (2005:580).

The variability of the women, the babies and the birthing environments were not recognised in the *data analysis* and all of the women were assigned a similar risk status. As Kitzinger (2005:79) notes, an experienced mother who is progressing in labour at 38 weeks with a baby whose weight is on the low side of normal is at relatively low risk. But the data analysis 'homogenised' both the participants and the interventions to produce a somewhat meaningless average form of care among an average population. For this reason, the findings of this trial are less than relevant to women and babies who are and whose birth environments are something other than 'average'.

Whereas the many aspects of this study may have tended towards the 'average', the *standard of practice* has been criticised for being somewhat less than that. In addition to the examples mentioned already, another is the way in which conservative management was taken to inappropriately non-interventionist extremes. This means that the insistence on minimal assistance to the birth of the aftercoming head is contrary to standard obstetric practice (Uotila et al, 2005). A further condemnation of the trial's low standard of obstetric practice emanates from Keirse who, *inter alia*, regrets that this trial continued for as long as it did. The continuation of the trial meant that the women and their babies were being deprived of the 'superior alternative' of external cephalic version (ECV) (2002:58). It is only possible to assume that ECV, to turn the baby to a cephalic presentation, was not attempted in order to ensure a suitable number of babies presenting by the breech.

Not unrelated to the criticism of the standard of practice is the problem of the *experience* of the attendants. In the protocol, the person assisting the vaginal breech birth is required 'to be skilled and experienced' in this mode of birth (Hannah et al, 2000). Drawing on her midwifery experience, Banks is critical of the absence of experienced clinicians at 2.6 per cent of the vaginal births. Of the allegedly 'skilled and experienced' obstetricians, though, the standard of expertise was such that instructions about how to deal with nuchal arms, footling breech and 'stuck head' needed to be posted on the TBT website (Banks, 2001).

This problem of lack of experience and expertise in the supremely important skill of assisting a breech birth is likely to be, yet again, associated with the sample size. Many of the participating centres were in countries where vaginal breech birth was certainly not the usual mode of breech delivery. Thus, if these centres were unable to contribute sufficient breech births, they would have had to withdraw from the trial. For this reason, many centres were required to 'triple their vaginal delivery rate overnight' (Kitzinger, 2005:79). Such an escalation certainly would not be able to ensure an experienced attendant at each vaginal breech birth. The result was that 18.5 per cent of vaginal breech births were assisted by an obstetrician in training, 2.9 per cent by a qualified midwife and one breech birth was attended only by a student midwife. Any astute observer would notice that, even though a caesarean is a far simpler technique than a breech birth, an obstetrician performed all but one of the planned caesareans. However, for only four out of five of the planned breech births was an obstetrician present (Keirse 2002:56).

In spite of this escalation in the proportion of breech births, it may be calculated that the average number of breech births in each centre may have been as low as six (Uotila et al, 2005). Clearly, such a low number makes it impossible to maintain even basic expertise in breech delivery. That the practitioners themselves were aware of their own deficiencies (Kotaska, 2004) may have aggravated their difficulties. The practitioners were encouraged to undertake breech deliveries when their usual caution dictated otherwise; that is they were being required to practise outwith their own comfort zone. This requirement, and the practitioners' obedience to it, may have been partly responsible for any less than satisfactory outcomes among the vaginal breech birth group.

In terms of the research *design*, the trial demonstrated more variation from the research protocol than would ordinarily be expected. The guidelines relating to the management of the aftercoming head were relaxed during the study period from 'no traction' to 'gentle traction while encouraging the mother to push' (Banks 2001:1). Obviously, such an alteration to the protocol is likely to call into question the consistency of the data.

As mentioned above (section 2.3), the importance of the scrupulous observation of *ethical principles* in the research process cannot be overstated. It has been suggested already that in the TBT ethical standards may have been allowed to slip; one example would be the tactics used to maintain the participating centres' motivation by offering them incentives for their involvement (Keirse, 2002:57). In his shrewd analysis, Keirse goes on to calculate the level of activity of the participating centres. Figures such as the number of births per annum are usually assumed to reflect the ability of a maternity unit to cope safely and effectively with more complicated and less common childbearing problems. That some of the participating centres may have been practising disconcertingly unsafely emerges from the calculation that the average number of term births per year (both breech and cephalic) was just 220. Thus, the overriding ethical principle of non-maleficence seems to have been disregarded (Thompson et al, 2006).

Another fundamental ethical principle which has been mentioned already and which is crucial to research as well as other aspects of health care, is fully informed consent. In the context of research it is good practice to allow the potential subject 24 to 48 hours' 'thinking time' or a 'cooling off period' between being given information about the study and being asked to consent to participation (AIMS/NCT, 1997). This allows the person time to contemplate on the implications of their involvement, to consult with their significant others and possibly to decide to refuse consent. Obviously, more time is preferable. An approach to seek consent from a potential participant at a stressful time, such as during labour or preoperatively, is to be deprecated. For this reason, one's heart sinks to read of the proportions of TBT participants who were recruited when they were in active labour. In the planned caesarean group 50 per cent of the women were recruited when they were already in labour. In the planned vaginal birth group this figure reached 83 per cent of the women. On this basis, it is necessary to question whether these women's consent could have been truly 'informed' and, hence, the entire ethical foundation of this trial.

The *time span* of the Term Breech Trial merits scrutiny, especially in view of the rapturous welcome and instant acceptance with which the findings were received by the obstetric fraternity. As mentioned already, the duration of the trial was foreshortened for less than convincing reasons. This reduced time span meant, though, that when the results were released (Hannah et al, 2000), the long-term data on maternal and neonatal morbidity were not available so could not be reported. It is possible that, if these data had been provided in that initial report, its reception and implementation would have been markedly different. This can be stated with confidence because, when these data were eventually published, they did not support the initial findings (Derrick, 2005; Whyte et al, 2004; Hannah et al, 2004). These later findings showed that there was, in fact, no difference between the two groups, either for the mothers or for their babies. Thus, conspiracy theorists might be forgiven for questioning the actual reason for the foreshortening of the trial.

The *conclusions* which may be drawn from the Term Breech Trial relate not only to whether a caesarean is the optimal form of care for a childbearing woman with a breech presentation, but also to the use of research in maternity care.

The value of this trial in assisting decisions about the care of the childbearing woman with a breech position is negligible. This statement is able to be made because the focus of any RCT is intended to be on one specific intervention. The Term Breech Trial, though, was not focused on a single intervention; it was not even focused on the multiplicity of optional interventions which contribute to the vaginal delivery of a baby by the breech. This trial served only to reflect the skills of a wide range of individual practitioners working in hugely differing environments with women and babies with little in common apart from a breech presentation at term. It may be argued that even the skills (or otherwise) of these practitioners may not be accurately reflected in the RCT reports; this is because those who were genuinely experienced were prevented by the research protocol from prudently exercising the judgement which they had learned from that experience. I venture to suggest that it is the exercise of prudent judgement, along with certain manual skills, which determine the success of a breech birth.

Further lessons may be drawn about the medical use of research. One of these lessons may be observed in the welcome extended to the TBT findings and the immediate effect on practice. It is totally inappropriate for practice to be changed simply on the basis of one study, even though it may be a large multicentre trial. The authority of the Cochrane Library lies in its development of a set of systematic reviews which have analysed groups of studies focusing on particular topics. These reviews will produce findings which demonstrate a number of points which are common to the groups of studies and which may be judged to be strong evidence. Thus, any single study should only be valued and implemented in relation to its contribution to a larger body of research evidence.

The powerful and influential agencies which ordinarily lead obstetric medical opinion were among those who initially welcomed the findings of the Term Breech Trial. Since the TBT 'emperor' has been shown to have 'no clothes', though, these professional leaders have maintained a stony silence which is strangely eloquent.

Not only has the TBT demonstrated the fallacious nature of medical claims to evidence-based practice, it may even have threatened the evidence base which it sought to expand. This is because the TBT has brought the RCT into disrepute by demonstrating all too clearly its shortcomings (Kotaska, 2004). The researchers, perhaps because they were not accustomed to vaginal breech birth, neglected to take account of the complexity of this mode of birth. Vaginal breech birth defies the one-dimensional approach inherent in the RCT. Thus, this trial has exposed the serious limitations of undertaking this form of research in an area as fraught with pitfalls and pratfalls as health care.

The doomsday scenario is presented by Keirse who, Cassandra-like, warns of the likely outcome if and when the medical practitioner continues to refuse to recognise that the TBT emperor really is naked. Keirse argues that the underlying purpose of this trial was to support the gradual medical progression towards, not only 'breech babies', but all babies being born by planned caesarean (2002:58). He, hopefully ironically, suggests that another RCT should be undertaken, along the lines of the Term Breech Trial. For this next RCT, though, the focus will be any form of vaginal birth. In this way he cynically suggests that the future of caesarean will be assured.

2.5.3 The research response to the Term Breech Trial

Other studies have been reported since the Term Breech Trial, which shed further light on the vexed problem of vaginal breech birth versus caesarean. The Finnish study by Uotila and colleagues (2005) surveyed a seven-year period. During this time, the only difference between the babies born by planned caesarean and those born by planned vaginal birth was the lower Apgar scores in the latter group. On the basis of these findings the authors argue in favour of vaginal breech births, but emphasise the importance of the attendant being part of a 'tradition' of this mode of birth (2005:582). Although these conclusions appear to be woman-friendly, they need careful interpretation. This is because of the exceptionally high quality of neonatal and infant care in Finland (Mander, in press) and also the fact that this was a retrospective, rather than a prospective survey. This research does, however, resonate with one of the weaknesses in the Term Breech Trial, in which the attendants lacked the necessary experience.

A study, which was undertaken in Austria, was somewhat more guarded in its support of vaginal breech birth (Krupitz et al, 2005). Although not statistically significant, this study found that serious neonatal morbidity featured more prominently among the planned vaginal birth group. As has already emerged as important, these researchers recognised the problem of the limited experience of the obstetricians in attending vaginal breech births. Krupitz and colleagues' guarded support of vaginal breech birth is circumscribed by a recommendation for complete information to be given to the woman about the risks.

2.6 Areas yet to be researched

In this chapter it has been shown that certain topics have been well addressed by research, although the quality of that research may leave something to be desired. I have also shown that some, particularly woman-related, areas are seriously in need of good research. Other, more specific topics have also been neglected by researchers.

2.6.1 The father and caesarean

The presence of the father has become an important aspect of childbirth in many westernised cultures (Mander, 2004a). Some features of his experience have been frequently and authoritatively examined by researchers. This research has shown the difficulties which the man encounters when he stays with his partner during her labour. Whether his difficulties have any effect on the woman's experience, the outcome of labour or the likelihood of caesarean has not been assessed. It is necessary to note, though, that the escalation in the number of caesareans parallels the entry and acceptance of the father into the birthing room (see section 1.3).

A potentially more easily researchable topic may be found in the experience of the couple or the father after the caesarean. The father's challenges certainly do not cease with the birth of the baby. It is uncertain, though, how the father whose partner has a caesarean is able to adjust to the multiplicity of events going on both within and around about him. These events may include the care of a traumatised partner and baby as well as his assumption of a range of other new roles. Not least among these is his role as a father. If appropriate help is to be provided for him, it is necessary to find out the basis of anecdotal reports that the father may return to work after his paternity leave with a sigh of relief.

2.6.2 The caesarean baby/child/person

The research on the well-being of the child born by caesarean tends to extend only into the very early months of the child's life. Less is known about this baby as she matures into a child and then into an independent person. What is known is that, in mythological terms, caesarean has been thought to convey particularly admirable attributes on the male child (see section 1.2.1). The fate of the girl child born by caesarean does not feature in the literature. These myths have led to caesarean being described as 'the godly way to enter the world' (Trolle, 1982:9). It is uncertain, though, what happens to these minor deities as they grow and mature into human beings.

These godly attributions probably derive from origins which are different from the modern 'Little emperors' (Mander, 2004b). The mode of birth, however, is the same. In China the one child policy has been enforced while, at the same time, the caesarean rate has far surpassed the western levels. The problems of the 'only children' resulting from the one child policy are becoming recognised as they enter their teenage and adult years. Little is known in the West, though, of the implications of caesarean birth for the developing person.

2.6.3 Economic aspects of caesarean

The economic argument in favour of caesarean is not infrequently added to those relating to convenience and maternal choice (Bost, 2003). The reality of the economic implications, though, is less straightforward. There is definitely a lack of strong research evidence about the relative costs of different modes of birth (Petrou et al, 2001). All too frequently the economic data, such as it is, originates in the USA. It is necessary to question the relevance of these data to countries where the health care system is, to say the least, different. The transfer of the economic debate across the Atlantic is even more difficult than transferring other phenomena. Thus, research into the economic aspects of caesarean must take account of cultural issues.

As the caesarean rates escalate, the need for such research becomes more urgent. This is not only to examine the argument that caesarean is justified on financial grounds. It is also necessary to find out to whom any costs accrue. The assumption that the costs are only to the health care system, through longer hospital stay and readmission, may need to be corrected to demonstrate the costs to the woman, her family and friends. These costs include not just financial costs, but also a range of emotional, social and opportunity costs. Further, to all of the costs of the 'index' pregnancy must be added those of any future pregnancy. These would include the financial and emotional costs attributable to any subsequent infertility investigations and the complications of childbearing (please see section 7.1.5).

2.7 Conclusion

In this chapter I have considered some of the main issues around research into caesarean. The problems with interpreting research have been addressed, together with factors which the critical reader of research should bear in mind. I have raised issues relating to the lack of research as well as to its limitations and to its non-use and misuse.

All of these issues have been brought together in an in-depth examination of the issues around the Term Breech Trial (see section 2.5.2). This trial has been shown to raise serious questions, not only for the childbearing woman and her baby, but also for practitioners in maternity and for researchers in general.

On the basis of the general condemnation of the Term Breech Trial and its findings, questions should be asked about the purpose of conducting this flawed study. Conspiracy theorists may be forgiven for assuming that the purpose of this trial was merely to reassure those already performing planned caesarean for breech presentation that they were right all along. The triumphalism with which the TBT findings were welcomed leads to anxiety that the jury may not just still be out on the issue of vaginal breech birth, but may actually have been discharged.

This pessimistic conclusion reflects the observations by Enkin (1992) who reports the response by Canadian physicians to encouragement to practice evidence-based medicine (EBM). Research evidence on the benefits and risks of caesarean was circulated to all medical practitioners working in the maternity field in Canada. The result was a minuscule drop in the caesarean rate (by 0.04 per cent per annum). Enkin attributes this abysmal response to physicians' reluctance to apply such findings to their own practice. He maintains that evidence which is 'international or even national in origin' (1992:217) is unlikely to be implemented unless local colleagues endorse its relevance. Thus, the physicians' own view of the evidence comes a poor third after local peer pressure and fear of litigation. To compound this dismal picture, Enkin suggests that such attitudes may not be amenable to educational interventions, but that financial incentives may be required in order to change obstetric practice.

3   The caesarean operation – issues and debates

The use of caesarean and its implications for all involved appropriately attracts much attention. Because of this, there is a tendency for the popular media to overlook matters relating to the operation itself. These surgery-related issues deserve attention for themselves as well as for their long-term effects and the light they shed on decision making. In this chapter I analyse the debates surrounding the actual caesarean operation, drawing on the research evidence where possible. I adopt a more or less chronological approach in presenting this material. Thus, the chapter begins with some discussion of the planning and timing of the operation, which obviously has serious consequences for the woman's degree of preparedness. The planning is clearly closely related to the indications for the caesarean, so the variability in rationale will emerge as an issue. The contribution of the woman *vis à vis* the different health care practitioners will be assessed. Because the incidence of secondary or repeat caesarean is crucial to the escalating caesarean rate, there will be an examination of the surgery-related factors which predispose to repeat caesarean. This chapter's chronological approach to the debates ends with consideration of issues relating to some of the surgical techniques involved in the operation itself.

3.1 Time factors

The timing of caesarean is important for a number of reasons. On the one hand, a planned surgical birth may be perceived by the woman as a way of taking control of the uncertainty about when the baby will be born. On the other hand, in an emergency, delay in the birth of the baby may be a cause of morbidity, or even mortality, if either the woman or the baby is in a seriously compromised condition.

3.1.1 Planning or not planning the caesarean

The decision that a caesarean should be undertaken is usually made following negotiation between the woman and her attendants (see Chapter 5). The timing of taking that decision by the various actors, though, will differ according to the circumstances. For example, a woman may decide before ever becoming pregnant that an uncomplicated vaginal birth is fundamentally important to her self-esteem and her vision of herself as a woman and mother. Whether and when she articulates this view to her attendants, though, will depend on when she is first in contact with them and on the quality of the relationship. Alternatively, an obstetrician may suspect during, for example, a woman's first labour that her pelvis is not large enough for an average sized baby to pass through it. Whether the obstetrician informs the woman of these suspicions may affect her plans for subsequent births.

In both of these examples, the decision is being made well in advance of the onset of labour. It is the start of labour which has traditionally determined the temporal classification of the caesarean. In the latter example, if a caesarean were to be eventually recommended and agreed, the surgery would be elective.

Then again, a problem which threatens the life of the woman and/or the baby may arise during the labour, such as serious antepartum haemorrhage. Such a problem might suggest that a caesarean would be appropriate. In these circumstances, this intrapartum operation would be regarded as an emergency procedure. In a small number of women, a condition may arise during pregnancy which means that an emergency caesarean is indicated.

In Scotland in 2004 the percentage of births by emergency caesarean had levelled off to 15.4 per cent (ISD, 2005b). If an optimistic view is taken, this levelling off may indicate a trend suggesting a decline in caesarean rates. Alternatively, it may be nothing more than a statistical artefact.

The percentage of births by elective caesarean in Scotland appears to be continuing its slow but inexorable rise, and reached 9.5 per cent in 2005 (ISD, 2005b). It may be, though, that this increase in the number of elective caesareans *per se* is of little significance. This is because such a large proportion of elective caesareans are undertaken as secondary operations following primary emergency operations. If the escalating caesarean rate is ever to be addressed, it should be by focusing on the emergency operations, rather than those performed electively.

This binary categorisation of elective or emergency surgery is not straightforward, though, and it may not be helpful. First, the word 'elective' is misleading. This is because the woman may assume that she is the only person to 'elect' or choose this form of birth. In fact, because this option is usually recommended to her, surgery is unlikely to be her choice alone.

The term 'emergency caesarean' is also misleading because it suggests that an immediately life-threatening condition exists. In reality, an emergency operation is any caesarean which is unplanned and is usually performed after the onset of labour. Whether the reason for the caesarean is actually immediately life threatening is quite another matter. All too often, the emergency operation may be performed at the behest of the partograph (see section 4.1) when the progress line falls below the action line, suggesting 'dystocia' or 'failure to progress'. In such circumstances, any threat is certainly not likely to be immediate.

To this complicated system of categorisation, needs to be added the 'emergency elective' operations. These happen when a woman, already destined for an elective operation, forestalls the surgeon by beginning to go into labour ahead of the date or time planned for surgery. Depending on the indications, an immediate operation may be thought necessary.

Because of this unsatisfactory and potentially misleading classification, new terminology has been proposed. One of these classifications is based on the findings of a two-stage survey involving 60 anaesthetists and 30 obstetricians (Lucas et al, 2000). These researchers recommend that the following clinical criteria should be used to classify caesareans:

1   immediate threat to life of mother and/or fetus
2   severe fetal and/or maternal compromise, but not life threatening
3   compromise responding to therapy, but the underlying problem persists
4   needing delivery, but no compromise is present
5   can be booked on an elective list (2000:348).

The advantages of this classification to professionals are clear. These authors do not, however, consider the possibility that such terminology may also help the mother to realise the seriousness or otherwise of her and her baby's condition.

In the course of a study of the responsiveness of maternity services, a more self-explanatory classification was developed (MacKenzie and Cooke, 2002). Although in this study it was only used for non-elective caesareans, this classification need not be exclusive:

- Crash – impending fetal death or serious maternal compromise anticipated (eg uterine rupture)
- Emergency – in labour evolving fetal distress, failing labour or maternal reasons
- Urgent – deteriorating fetal and/or maternal health before the onset of labour
- Pre-empted – condition arising before the onset of labour or rupture of membranes (2002:499).

MacKenzie and Cooke's categorisation appears to lack the precision of the one prepared by Lucas and colleagues, while retaining the potential for inducing panic. The RCOG Sentinel Audit report features all the advantages of both of these categorisations (Thomas and Paranjothy, 2001). By omitting category 3 from the classification by Lucas and colleagues, it retains their precision, while achieving MacKenzie and Cooke's brevity.

3.1.2 Implementing the decision in an emergency

In the case of the most life-threatening situations, speedy intervention becomes crucial. These are the 'crash' caesareans (MacKenzie and Cooke, 2002) and Lucas and colleagues' 'category 1' situations. The optimum time within which the baby should be born in these circumstances has been quite arbitrarily set at 30 minutes maximum. This time period is the 'decision-to-delivery' interval, which was investigated by Helmy and colleagues (2002). These researchers attempted to evaluate the feasibility of this 30-minute standard. They undertook a series of surveys in a well-staffed labour ward with an integral operating department. In the first baseline survey, in only 26 out of 73 caesareans (36 per cent) was the baby born within 30 minutes of the decision being taken. On the basis of this disconcertingly poor result, a 'time sheet' was introduced into the woman's medical notes. This document was used to record the time the anaesthetist, operating department attendant and paediatrician were called and arrived. The authors claim that this 'time sheet' improved the subsequent performance, which shows a definite trend to reduce the interval from decision to delivery. This project demonstrates that 'naming, shaming and blaming' staff may still be an effective way of persuading them to 'drop everything and run'.

As well as this blame culture, certain other details in the study by Helmy and colleagues merit closer attention. The focus on documentation in this 'audit' matters, because it was the new paperwork which, it is claimed, was responsible for reducing the interval times. In the authors' account of factors responsible for the delays, 'poor note keeping' and anaesthetic-related issues predominate. Whether some interdisciplinary difficulties are present in this clinical area can only be surmised.

Another point which remains unexplained in this research is the large proportion of caesareans performed under general anaesthesia. In the data provided 18 out of 26 women (69 per cent) were given a general anaesthetic, 6 (23 per cent) had a spinal anaesthetic and 2 (8 per cent) had an epidural anaesthetic. It is necessary to question the rationale for such a large proportion of general anaesthetics being administered. This form of anaesthesia is reputedly quicker than regional anaesthesia. This benefit, however, must be viewed alongside general anaesthesia's increased risks for both mother and baby (see section 3.3.1.6). It is necessary to question whether these researchers were seeking to reduce the time interval at all costs and with little regard for the welfare of the mother and baby.

A reduction of the decision-to-delivery interval was also one of the findings in another study into this aspect of quality of care (MacKenzie and Cooke, 2002). These researchers collected data prospectively without clinicians' knowledge, using the urgency scale mentioned above (see section 3.1.1). There is no mention of whether ethical approval was sought or obtained. For 'crash' caesareans (n=22), a mean time for the decision-to-delivery interval of 27.4 minutes was achieved.

While regretting that the time interval has not been reduced since previous data collections in 1989 and 1996, MacKenzie and Cooke note the reduction in the time interval for caesareans for fetal distress performed between 02.00 and 07.00. This improvement happened in spite of reduced night time staffing. The authors attribute this effect to the absence of 'planned' caesareans and inductions of labour. Unsurprisingly, Robinson (2002) suggests that if operating departments were not overburdened with these planned interventions, the delays in what appear to be urgent and necessary operations could probably be reduced. It is these delays which are responsible for morbidity and possibly mortality and for this reason, if for no other, the delays need to be reduced.

The classification debate was applied to the issue of the decision-to-delivery interval by the RCOG Sentinel Audit report (Thomas and Paranjothy, 2001:56). This report argues that the classification should be used to make communication more effective in emergencies. This would mean that the classification would impress on potentially recalcitrant colleagues the urgency of the situation. While effective communication is highly desirable, it is difficult to surmise how effective such a strategy would be in motivating diverse disciplinary groups to work as a team.

The decision-to-delivery interval is clearly crucial in genuine emergency situations. To understand what is meant by 'emergency', appropriate terminology needs to be introduced and employed. These factors are closely interrelated and have serious implications for women and babies, as well as for health care providers. It is necessary to bear in mind, though, the policy implications of these interrelated issues. These implications relate to the widespread assumption of the safety of hospital birth, which is attributed to the easy and constant availability of personnel to deal with life-threatening situations for the woman and/or baby. These studies show that this 'rescue operation' is unlikely to be able to be performed in less than 30 minutes; these findings must cast doubt on the policy of routinely admitting women into hospital to labour and to give birth. Of course, calculations of the decision-to-delivery interval assume that the relevant staff are available on the hospital premises. This assumption may not always hold true, as in a situation when I diagnosed a prolapsed cord in a first time mother in early labour. In this genuinely life-threatening emergency, the anaesthetist who was supposedly on call was found to have left the hospital site to go shopping. Fortunately, the baby was eventually born in a good condition.

3.2 Indications for performing a caesarean

In an ideal world where evidence-based knowledge is available and applied, the reasons or indications for performing a caesarean would be fixed, immutable and unchanging across time and continents. Perhaps unfortunately that ideal world does not yet exist. This means that the indications for performing a caesarean vary according to a number of factors. Some of these factors may be explicit, but many are unspoken and may also be unrecognised. I venture to suggest that some of these factors involve the development of knowledge and technological and other skills; an example would be the factors underpinning some obstetricians' enthusiasm for all 'breech babies' to be born by caesarean (please see section 2.5.2). Other factors may be put down to matters as frivolous as whims of fashion. The question of whose fashion, though, is a matter which has still to be addressed.

The interpretation and interaction of the various indications for the caesarean operation is complex. This means that the indications for caesarean develop their own dynamic. This is a dynamism which is subject to many influences, and the result is a change in the threshold at which the operation will be performed. A familiar example may be found in recent history, in the high maternal mortality rates associated with general anaesthesia for caesarean (Mander, 1993a). In the late 1960s anaesthetic problems caused caesarean to be seriously risky, especially for the woman (see section 3.3.1.6), so the operation tended to be strenuously avoided. With the advent of epidural analgesia, though, this particular risk was lowered and so, correspondingly, was the threshold for performing the caesarean operation. The lowering of this major barrier made way for the escalating caesarean rates with which we are now familiar. In this example the risk was to the mother's life; a current and ongoing example of risk to the baby may be found in the debate over the optimal mode of birth for babies presenting by the breech (see section 2.5.2).

These indications need a further level of 'interpretation', because the enthusiasm of the various participants for the operation (as well as their level of skill) needs to be taken into account (see Chapter 5). This, like the categorisation of urgency mentioned in section 3.1.1, serves to limit the value of 'absolute' criteria and to make many of the indications more 'relative'. Similarly, this variability in enthusiasm would also affect whether the caesarean, if it became necessary, was an elective or an emergency operation. The gravity of the condition, for example maternal hypertension, would also influence the urgency of the situation, meaning that the same condition could be an indication for either an elective or an emergency caesarean.

In this part of the book, I focus on the most standard health-related factors which are used to justify caesareans. The more social and societal aspects, such as the woman's choice, are addressed elsewhere in Chapters 5, 8 and 9.

3.2.1 The indications: who benefits?

In order to outline the indications for caesarean it is helpful to consider who is intended to be the main beneficiary from the operation being performed. The usual beneficiaries would be either the woman or the baby or both. The frequency of the reasons or indications for caesarean may be helpful to give an impression of their importance. To do this I draw on the data provided by MacKenzie and Cooke (2002).

3.2.1.1 Woman-related factors

Placenta praevia is widely regarded as an absolute indication for caesarean (Penn and Ghaem-Maghami, 2001), but even this potential threat to the woman's life should be considered carefully. Caution is urged in view of the changing dimensions of the uterus towards the end of pregnancy. So minor degrees of placenta praevia (grades 1–2), if the baby's head is engaged, present a relatively low level of risk. Of course, also due to the changing uterine dimensions, an ultrasound scan in early pregnancy showing a marked degree of placenta praevia may be irrelevant or misleading near term.

Dystocia or unsatisfactory (progress in) labour is not purely woman-related, there are indubitably fetal factors too. A diagnosis of 'dystocia' is likely to be made by use of a partograph. Therefore, this highly subjective diagnosis raises a multitude of questions, some of which are addressed in Chapter 4. Caesarean, though an easy answer, may not always be the correct one (Glantz and McNanley, 1997). In approximately 53 per cent of emergency caesareans, dystocia is the major indication. The unfortunate term 'failure to progress' is another alternative name.

3.2.1.2 Factors relating to the baby

Fetal distress (or compromise) is another term which is too imprecise to be of help. The method of diagnosis of any distress and the stage of labour are but two of the factors which need to be taken into account when contemplating the possibility of caesarean. Although routine continuous electronic fetal monitoring (CEFM) is widely used to provide early warning of fetal distress, its value has yet to be firmly established (Thacker et al, 2001). Approximately one third of emergency caesareans are undertaken for fetal distress.

Cord prolapse or cord presentation may also be regarded as absolute indications for caesarean. These, however, are other situations in which the level of the baby's head and the stage of labour are likely to influence any decision about how the baby should be born.

Breech presentation is another possible indication for caesarean which is highly contentious. Possibly due to declining obstetric skills combined with increasing obstetric fears of litigation, many women may not be presented with any alternative to a caesarean birth (Hofmeyr and Hannah, 2003). Approximately 6 per cent of emergency caesareans are for malpresentation. (Please see section 2.5.2.)

The mode of birth of a low birth weight baby will be determined by factors such as any degree of compromise, the gestational age and the presentation. Again, the situation is far from clear-cut.

The rationale for a caesarean being performed for a multiple pregnancy varies according to factors including the presentation of the babies, their number, their size, their gestational age and any compromise.

3.2.1.3 Factors relating to the woman and the baby

Placental abruption, because of the threats which it poses to both fetal and maternal health, is well nigh an absolute indication for caesarean. This diktat may need to be moderated, though, by the extent of the abruption and, thus, the conditions of woman and baby.

Cephalo-pelvic disproportion, with or without macrosomia, may not be diagnosed definitively until the woman is in labour, although the weight of any previous babies may helpfully indicate the size of her pelvis. Approximately 7 per cent of emergency caesareans are for this reason.

If the baby is in a transverse lie, that is a shoulder presentation, whether a vaginal birth is possible is dependent on the size of the woman's pelvis and the size/gestation of the baby. The complications, though, mean that the woman may justifiably be discouraged from attempting a vaginal birth.

3.2.2 Issues around the operation

For a woman who has never had a caesarean previously, the operation may be termed a *primary* caesarean. Inevitably, therefore, if she has already undergone a previous caesarean, any subsequent operation would be a *secondary* or repeat operation. Many of the issues relating to the primary or secondary nature of the operation are linked to the VBAC debate and are addressed in Chapter 8. The factors which influence the VBAC decision, though, have their origins in the earlier caesarean. It is, therefore, necessary to explore here those surgery-related factors and their implications.

Irrespective of the skin incision, which is ordinarily a 'Pfannensteil' or 'bikini line' incision, it is almost invariably followed by a horizontal incision into the lower part (or segment) of the woman's uterus or womb (Mathai and Hofmeyr, 2003). This lower segment incision is preferred on the grounds that the blood supply and uterine activity are reduced in this lower area. This means that, supposedly, the risk of haemorrhage from the uterine wound is reduced and healing is facilitated respectively. Occasionally, a 'classical' or vertical incision into the upper segment of the uterus may need to be employed. Although this form of incision carries certain benefits, they may be outweighed by the additional risks.

Following the birth of the baby and the placenta, the incision into the uterus and the superficial tissues will be repaired by suturing. The repair to the uterus may be made separately, in two or more layers, or in a single layer. The materials and techniques which are used will vary according to a number of factors.

Following the operation, healing proceeds in the damaged tissues, as it does following any form of bodily hurt. This is of particular importance in the uterine wound, as the effectiveness of healing is said to affect subsequent childbearing. In general terms, the adequacy of healing has been shown to be determined by factors such as age, hydration, cleanliness, freedom from infection, certain medications, tissue oxygenation and nutrition (RCSE, 2003). Clearly, in a childbearing woman these factors will ordinarily function healthily to ensure that her wound heals optimally and securely.

The healing of the uterine wound, as happens with any wound, involves a healthy localised inflammatory reaction. Platelets and thrombin in the wound form a network with collagen fibres. Cells such as macrophages are carried to the wound site and fibroblasts develop to facilitate healing and the formation of a scar (Ganong, 1997). In this way, the integrity or wholeness of the uterus is re-established.

Under certain circumstances, though, the edges of a wound which was thought to have healed may begin to separate or undergo 'dehiscence', possibly leading to rupture. These circumstances may include 'marked distension' (Brunner and Suddarth, 1992:150). In the context of the caesarean operation, this separation may occasionally occur in a subsequent pregnancy or labour due to distension and contractions. This separation constitutes an obstetric accident known as 'rupture of the uterus', which carries serious risks for the baby and for the mother. In this event the baby's oxygen supply could be severely compromised, which could result in damage to the baby or possibly death. Under such circumstances, the mother might die due to haemorrhage or other complications. Alternatively, she might encounter such serious bleeding or damage to her uterus as to warrant it being removed surgically by hysterectomy.

On the basis of these potential problems, the question arises of the number of caesareans which a woman may undergo. This question is difficult to answer in absolute terms. It is sufficient to say here that the risks associated with the surgery, the anaesthetic and the recovery period have been shown to increase with the number of caesareans an individual woman undergoes (Dodd et al, 2004).

3.3 Surgery-related issues

It may be assumed that once the caesarean decision has been agreed, then the operation is straightforward, even to the point of being routine. This is far from the case. There are a number of alternatives for a number of issues; in some of which decision making may be assisted by research evidence. I consider these issues here in chronological order.

3.3.1 Psychological preparation for the operation

Depending on the time frame, the woman will have more or less time available in which to complete her physical and psychological preparation. If there is more time, this preparation is likely to involve her gathering information from a range of sources, such as suitably experienced family and friends, childbirth educators, bookshops and libraries and, of course, the internet. Stewart recognises the web's frequent use by childbearing women and traces the development of e-health. She considers the implications of clients' internet use for health care providers (2001; 2005). She identifies staff misgivings that their 'all-knowing' (2001:13) status will be jeopardised and shows how these misgivings carry the potential for damage to their relationship with the client. Existing advice for medical personnel about how to cope with internet-literate patients is shown to be applicable to midwifery clients. Stewart's analysis of internet use is surprisingly positive, leading the reader to wonder whether there may actually be some valuable material on the internet.

3.3.1.1 Hospitalisation

It may appear unnecessary to state that a woman needs to be admitted to a tertiary level health care facility if a caesarean is to be performed. This admission may be for an elective caesarean or may involve an emergency transfer from a secondary level facility.

The link between admission to a maternity hospital for the birth and undergoing a caesarean, though, is even less straightforward than other aspects. The environment of the labour has profound effects on the mode of birth which may not be easily explained. These effects appear to make a caesarean more likely if the woman has already been hospitalised. This complex issue is clearly exemplified by one study which showed that planning to give birth at home is associated with a 50 per cent reduction in the incidence of both assisted birth and caesarean (Chamberlain et al, 1997). Thus, admission to hospital appears to not only present a solution to a problem, but also to be part of that problem.

3.3.1.2 Fasting

Since the middle of the twentieth century the link between caesarean and the limitation of oral intake during labour has become stronger and the resulting protocols more strictly followed. A vicious cycle of all women being treated as being at risk for the sake of a small number with bad outcomes began with the identification of aspiration pneumonitis (Mendelson, 1946). Working in a setting where general anaesthesia was widely used for relatively healthy childbirth, this research identified the dangers of the woman regurgitating and aspirating acid stomach contents into her lungs during obstetric general anaesthesia. Far from being a common problem, aspiration pneumonitis has subsequently been attributed to unsatisfactory anaesthetic techniques (Johnson et al, 1989), possibly by inadequately skilled 'anaesthesiologists'. Pharmacological approaches to resolving this problem are addressed below (please see section 3.3.1.6).

Working on the logical premise that a full stomach must contain acidic material, the obvious conclusion was drawn that an empty stomach would contain nothing. Hence, there would be no risk of aspiration pneumonitis, should a general anaesthetic become necessary. Even though logical, this approach is unable to ensure either an empty stomach or that any contents are less acid (Johnson et al, 1989). These problems appear to be aggravated by delayed stomach emptying due to narcotic analgesic medication to control labour pain (Broach and Newton, 1988).

Mendelson's syndrome has been shown to be preventable during intubation by the use of cricoid pressure (Sellick's manoeuvre) and a cuffed endotracheal tube (Dresner and Freeman, 2001). Crawford (1986) argued that the dangers of aspiration pneumonitis did not actually predate women being denied oral intake in labour. These dangers appear to have been only exacerbated by the routine administration in labour of antacids, such as magnesium trisilicate. Thus, a virtuous cycle intended to make caesarean safer was transformed into an iatrogenic cycle.

The implications for practice of this cycle have been researched in Australia; midwives whose experience is only in hospitals may be more likely to accept the fasting doctrine than midwives who have other experience (Parsons, 2004). This researcher emphasises that eating and drinking bring the woman, not only nutritional, but also personal and psychological benefits: '[women in labour] need to feel that they have some control, and may feel nauseated or dehydrated if not allowed to do what their body is telling them to do' (Respondent R66UH, Parsons, 2004:79).

As well as the lack of any established benefit of fasting in labour in case of an emergency caesarean, attitudes to fasting prior to elective surgery, such as caesarean, are also changing. The routine of preoperative fasting, like withholding oral intake in labour, aims to reduce both the quantity and the acidity of the stomach contents; again the intention is to reduce or minimise any harm caused by regurgitation and aspiration. The orthodoxy requires that the 'patient' should have 'nil by mouth' from midnight prior to surgery (Brady et al, 2003). Because of the difficulty in organising an operating department to function punctually, surgery is invariably delayed; so a fast of, supposedly, eight or nine hours may extend to fifteen to eighteen hours. As well as serious anxiety, such an extension causes a range of adverse metabolic changes.

In their review of the existing research, Brady and colleagues (2003) find that a shorter period of fluid restriction causes no greater perioperative morbidity than a longer fluid fast. On the contrary, allowing water to drink preoperatively is found to be associated with a significantly lower quantity of gastric secretions. These researchers implicitly recognise the medical adherence to traditional orthodoxy when they generously observe that, despite the research evidence, 'Practice has been slow to change' (Brady et al, 2003:1).

As well as fasting prior to the caesarean operation, another orthodoxy has been the withholding of oral fluids and food postoperatively, until bowel activity is known to have resumed. The rationale has been that the resumption of bowel activity may be impaired by oral intake, bringing the spectre of intestinal obstruction (paralytic ileus) (please see section 6.1.2.3). A systematic review found that an early intake of oral fluids and food is not associated with any increase in nausea, vomiting, delayed bowel movement/passage of flatus or paralytic ileus (Mangesi and Hofmeyr, 2002). The reviewers found quite the reverse, that early oral intake is linked with earlier resumption of bowel activity, reduced postoperative hospital stay and less abdominal distension. The conclusion may safely be drawn that, far from delaying recovery, early intake may actually facilitate a return to normal gastro-intestinal and other functioning.

3.3.1.3 Hair removal

In the era of the 'Brazilian' when the removal of pubic hair has become a fashion statement, it may seem surprising that hair removal prior to surgery remains an issue. The traditional view that body hair must be removed from any intended wound site is said to have been based on the logical assumption that hair is not sterile. Therefore, in the interests of wound cleanliness and healing, it has long been required that hair should be removed, usually by means of some kind of razor.

In the area of general surgery, the fallacy of this argument has been clearly demonstrated (Tanner et al, 2003). Because a razor is dragged over the skin to remove hair, any irregularities in the skin are abraded, causing microscopic cuts. It seems likely that pathogenic organisms enter these damaged areas, thus contaminating the site and causing postoperative wound infection. Additionally, any serous exudate from the damaged areas provides an ideal culture medium for the further growth of pathogenic organisms.

Thus, in an attempt to reduce the incidence of wound infection, this problem has attracted considerable research attention in the general surgical area. Tanner and colleagues (2003) recount the attempts to reduce wound infections by limiting the damage to skin in the area of the wound. These attempts include the use of clippers which cut the hair close to the patient's skin. A short stubble remains and skin damage is reduced. An alternative agent is depilatory creams, which remove hairs by dissolving them. To do this, though, the cream must be in contact with the hair for long enough to dissolve it, which may take up to 20 minutes. The chemical agents in depilatories carry a risk of allergic and skin reactions; thus, a time-consuming skin test is a wise precaution. A further question of who removes the hair needs to be addressed; the patient or client may be perfectly able to complete this task satisfactorily (Tanner et al, 2003).

In the maternity area, the fashion for removing pubic/perineal hair began, coincidentally, with the invention of the safety razor in the opening years of the twentieth century (Drayton, 1990:32). The practice of reducing the female genitalia to an apparently pre-pubescent state during the 'preparation' for labour has been challenged virtually ever since, and has been abandoned in many settings. The challenges have been on the grounds of infection risks, discomfort during regrowth and feelings of violation at being subjected to such a humiliating experience. The ground-breaking research by Mona Romney (1980) crucially endorsed these challenges, by showing no benefit in routinely removing pubic/perineal hair by either shaving or partially shaving. Subsequent research showed that, as has been observed elsewhere, 'practice was slow to change' (Garforth and Garcia, 1987). On the basis of their systematic review, Basevi and Lavender (2000) found that in terms of the mother's health and satisfaction and the baby's health, there is no evidence to support routine pubic/perineal shaving as a preparation for labour.

The question arises of the extent to which these findings are able to be extrapolated to the woman undergoing a caesarean. The crucial difference is that this woman will definitely have a wound and a scar, whereas this is far from certain for a woman embarking on labour. Further, the Pfannensteil (transverse suprapubic) incision is invariably made on or below the pubic hair line. The research on pre-operative hair removal prior to caesarean appears to be meagre. The topic of shaving manifested itself in two studies seeking to address the problem of post-caesarean wound infections. An earlier study found that hair removal methods had no significant effect on infection rates, although some of the data needed to be re-analysed (Moir-Bussy et al, 1985). A Danish study, on the other hand, demonstrated that wound infection rates could be reduced by a package of measures including cutting the pubic hair rather than shaving it off (Frost et al, 1989). A New Zealand study of 'preparation' for caesarean has demonstrated a marked reduction in the number of wound infections (Calvert and Stinson, in press). The midwife researchers implemented a package of skin preparation measures, including clipping the pubic hair and a preoperative shower sponge. It is paradoxical to note that, while practice in general surgery is changing and midwifery practice has changed, obstetric practice remains firmly entrenched in the early days of the twentieth century when Mr Gillette first patented his safety razor.

3.3.1.4 Bladder catheterisation

The practice of inserting an indwelling catheter into the woman's bladder prior to caesarean is so widespread as to be routine. The rationale for this invasive procedure is mainly to reduce the risk of damage to the bladder during surgery (Page et al, 2003). It should be added, though, that because of the close adherence of the bladder to the anterior wall of the lower segment, a distended bladder would impede the operation. Some would further argue that there may be advantages, assuming that the catheter remains in position postoperatively, in the woman not being required to move about excessively to allow her to pass urine. Additionally, it has been suggested that the catheter prevents over-distension of the bladder, thus minimising the risk of long-term problems with bladder function.

As well as these possible advantages, as with any intervention, there are disadvantages. On an anecdotal basis, some women find the idea of the catheter unpleasant, as a foreign body, and other women may feel it to be physically uncomfortable. More authoritative evidence is discussed by Thomas (2000) in relation to American data on 'Hospital Acquired Infections' (HAIs). In an attempt to minimise the media feeding frenzy associated with these iatrogenic conditions, they have been 're-branded' as 'Health Care Associated Infections' (DoH, 2005a). While this change in name may deflect the blame away from hospitals, it does nothing to reduce the impact of these conditions.

On the basis of American data, Thomas shows that a large majority (66 per cent) of HAIs are linked with intravenous drips or urinary catheters. She goes on to argue that women who undergo a caesarean have at least two of the major risk factors for developing an HAI. These are a surgical wound and a urinary catheter. She extrapolates that 4,000 UK women will develop an infection because of having had a caesarean.

Thus, it is apparent that the benefits of urinary catheterisation, outlined above, should be regarded with some degree of caution.

3.3.1.5 Medication

As mentioned already (see section 3.3.1.2), should a general anaesthetic be necessary for a caesarean, the risk of aspiration pneumonitis materialises. Fasting has been widely recommended and imposed in an attempt to reduce this risk. With the falling number of elective caesareans under general anaesthesia, the need for a quick acting measure to reduce both the risk of acid aspiration and, should it happen, the effects, has increased. A range of prophylactic measures have been introduced, including antacids, H_2 receptor antagonists, proton pump inhibitors and prokinetic agents.

While antacids are effective in making the stomach contents less acid, they also increase their volume, which may serve to outweigh any possible benefits. Two groups of drugs, whose effectiveness is greater than the antacids, are the H_2 receptor antagonists, of which ranitidine is a widely used example, and the proton pump antagonists, such as omeprazole. These agents serve to not only make the stomach contents less acid, but also reduce the quantity of the gastric secretions (Paranjothy et al, 2004).

3.3.1.6 The anaesthetic

As I have indicated already in this chapter, *general anaesthesia* for caesarean carries certain risks (please see section 3.3.1.2 above). To these should be added the increased risk of failure of intubation in a childbearing woman, which are increased if the surgery is an emergency (Dresner and Freeman, 2001; Coyle, 1992). These risks constitute the major reasons why regional anaesthesia is superseding general anaesthesia for caesarean. Other factors, though, such as the woman being awake and retaining some degree of involvement, or even control, in the birth, may also make regional anaesthesia more attractive to her.

The major advantage of general anaesthesia relates, assuming it goes smoothly, to its speed. Thus, depending on the anaesthetic skills available, it is only likely to be recommended in situations where the condition of the woman and/or the baby is seriously compromised and an immediate birth is a priority. The risks of general anaesthesia are associated with some of the physiological changes of advanced pregnancy, which may cause difficulty in the induction of the general anaesthetic. These changes include supine hypotension, when the pregnant woman lies on her back and the weight of the uterus and its contents interferes with the return of blood to the woman's heart and lungs. Both her and her baby's oxygen supply are likely to be impeded. Additionally, the physiological changes which make heartburn a common problem in pregnancy, also make the contents of the stomach more likely to be regurgitated and aspired into the lungs (please see section 3.3.1.2 above). Of course, the majority of the drugs which are administered to the woman intravenously will cross the placenta and, if given time, have a similar effect on the baby as on the woman.

It may be assumed, in view of these risks, that a woman's request for a general anaesthetic might be questioned, or at least discussed. It is my observation that this is not invariably the case. One reason for a woman requesting a caesarean under general anaesthesia is said to be *needle phobia* (Dennis, 1994). The authoritative literature about needle phobia is scant. This diagnosis does appear, however, to be used as an indication for caesarean under general anaesthesia.

From the point of view of my experience as a midwife, I find it difficult to imagine how a woman could undergo any kind of caesarean without encountering a number of needles for fluid administration as well as intravenous and other kinds of injections. The nature of the needle phobia in these circumstances is sometimes unclear. In a case study, the woman's phobia related essentially to the pain of any injections, and when the pain was addressed her care progressed relatively uneventfully (Dennis, 1994). On the other hand, Koppel and Thapar list a litany of incapacitating symptoms characteristic of needle phobia (1998). This leads to the conclusion that, although the pain of injections may be an important feature of needle phobia, there are other components, which may be amenable to psychological and/or psychiatric intervention.

The problems of general anaesthesia for the woman having a caesarean do not end with the induction of the anaesthetic. A condition which has a 'classical association' with caesarean (Lyons and Akerman, 2005:35) is *awareness*. Sometimes known as 'intra-operative awareness', this condition has been defined as 'failure of general anaesthesia to render a patient insensate' (Osterman et al, 2001:198). Awareness means that the woman retains a sufficient degree of consciousness, in spite of her general anaesthetic, for her to be able to recognise her situation and events going on around her. While the woman retains some sensory function, her motor function has ordinarily been removed, so she is unable to alert those around her to her level of consciousness.

This disconcerting condition, which has long been recognised as a problem during caesarean, derives from an imbalance between the maternal and fetal/ neonatal needs (Lyons and Akerman, 2005). On the one hand the mother requires an effective anaesthetic, while the neonate needs to be alert and uncompromised by anaesthetic medication. Various cocktails of drugs have been introduced in an attempt to overcome awareness. The drug regime used is recommended to be determined by the neonatal resuscitation facilities available. In the absence of good neonatal facilities it has been argued that the fetal condition should be prioritised, in that awareness should not be the 'driving concern' (Lyons and Akerman, 2005:35).

Occasionally, the woman with awareness may retain some degree of motor function, as in the case of one woman whose caesarean I attended. This was an incident which happened at a very early stage in my midwifery career, so the seriousness of this problem impressed itself on me profoundly. The woman was having a caesarean under general anaesthesia for prolonged labour due to a pre-viously undiagnosed pelvic malformation. As the obstetrician began to make the skin incision, the woman moved her hand towards the incision site, presumably in an unconscious but futile attempt to push away the scalpel. The operating theatre became deafeningly silent and everyone froze momentarily until the anaesthetist achieved a more suitable level of anaesthesia.

Although I was unable to follow her up this woman may have been one of those who have been found to experience post traumatic stress disorder (PTSD; Osterman et al, 2001). These North American researchers recruited a volunteer sample of 16 people who reported having experienced awareness. There were ten controls. A majority of the awareness group and none of the controls met the diagnostic criteria for suffering from PTSD at the time of a structured interview. The awareness group included three women who had experienced awareness while undergoing a caesarean, which had been performed between 36 and 22 years previously. These women's recollections were described in the following terms:

> Subject 13   Felt she was dying, couldn't breathe, heard doctors comment on her blue colour of her nails, heard their panic, felt terror, helpless.

> Subject 10   Felt skin being cut, felt unsafe, terror, paralysis, heard talking and laughing.

> Subject 16   Felt restrained, helpless, felt unsafe, felt her doctors did not care, gurgling noises and talking.
>
> (Osterman et al, 2001:201)

Thus, it appears that awareness due to inadequate general anaesthesia may be a cause of PTSD. Whether there are any other reasons for PTSD associated with caesarean is discussed in section 7.1.2.

Having examined the situation regarding general anaesthesia for caesarean, it is now necessary to consider the alternative, regional anaesthesia, which includes epidural analgesia/anaesthesia, spinal anaesthesia and combined spinal epidural (CSE) anaesthesia. It has been argued that spinal anaesthesia is preferable on the grounds that otherwise the 'strong sensations of pulling and discomfort' are a source of complaints (Dresner and Freeman, 2001:136). For this reason, it is recommend that, unless an epidural has been functioning exceptionally well during labour, a spinal anaesthetic should be introduced.

The major issue for regional anaesthesia is the relationship between it and cae-sarean. In an authoritative systematic review, the main benefit of regional analgesia is shown to be that it also serves, when necessary, as an anaesthetic:

> A functioning epidural allows the option of regional anaesthesia for inter-ventions such as caesarean section or manual removal of retained placenta, thereby avoiding the risks associated with general anaesthesia.
>
> (Anim-Somuah et al, 2005)

Thus, an intervention intended to relieve pain in labour may also serve as an anaesthetic to permit an 'emergency' caesarean. The question which arises, though, is whether regional analgesia increases the likelihood of a caesarean being required. It has long been recognised that the use of regional analgesia may influence the course of labour. Obstetric anaesthetists, however, have fought long and hard to refute any suggestion that their provision of pain control accelerates the 'cascade of intervention' (please see section 1.4.9). This vicious cycle may be associated with persistent malposition of the fetal head, prolonged labour, increased use of oxytocin and with instrumental or operative birth. The conclusion reached by Anim-Somuah and colleagues' systematic review, however, is that having a regional analgesia does not increase the likelihood of caesarean for 'dystocia' or prolonged labour. This review does, though, demonstrate an increased likelihood of caesarean for fetal distress; such compromise may be the fetal response to the use of oxtocic drugs to accelerate a labour which has been inadvertently artificially slowed by the use of regional analgesia.

3.3.2 The surgery

It may be assumed that the details of the operation have few implications for the woman or for non-medical personnel. This assumption fails to recognise the impor-tance of effective healing, particularly of the uterine wound, for future childbearing. For this reason, it is helpful to consider certain aspects of the surgery itself.

The type of skin incision is currently subject to little debate. The Pfannensteil or 'bikini line' incision, although requiring greater surgical skills and causing heav-ier blood loss, is cosmetically more acceptable and, hence, universally preferred when time permits.

In the event of a subsequent pregnancy it is crucial that any previous uterine wound should be completely and strongly healed (see Chapter 8). This means that the suturing of that wound after the caesarean birth is considered fundamentally important. The method used to suture the wound in the uterus has attracted some research attention. This is because the 'traditional' method has been to repair the wound in two layers. This method has involved, first, a single continuous inter-locking suture, rather like a blanket stitch. The second, similar, layer of suturing effectively 'buries' the first layer.

An innovative method, involving only the first layer in a single layer, has been introduced in North America. This innovation carries short-term benefits and cost savings; first because of a reduction in the time each woman spends in the operating theatre and, second, because of the availability of the operating theatre for other operations (O'Brien-Abel, 2003). There was an attempt to evaluate the effects of this innovative method (Bujold et al, 2002). Subsequent rupture of the uterus was the criterion for evaluation. In order to assess the birth outcomes following repair using these two methods, these researchers undertook a retrospective survey of women's medical notes for the previous 12 years.

Bujold and colleagues found that rupture of the uterus happened in 8 (0.54 per cent) of the 1,491 women in whom the traditional double layer method had been used. For the women in whom the innovative single layer method had been used, however, the risk of rupture of the uterus was significantly higher at 3.1 per cent (15 out of 489 women). Thus, these researchers consider that, in the long term, single layer closure is significantly riskier than the traditional technique. It is not clear why this should be. There may be increased strength of the scar resulting from a repair in two layers, or due to the better approximation of the tissues or to the more adequate blood supply. The nature of the suture material which is used to repair the caesarean wound may affect its healing (Dodd et al, 2003:5). While this suggestion is eminently reasonable, I have been unable to locate any research literature examining this issue.

3.3.3 Present or absent?

The personnel who are present in the operating theatre during a caesarean are kept to a minimum. This is partly because of the risks of infection being introduced, partly to reduce staff costs and partly to maintain as personal an atmosphere as possible for the birth. If students or other observers are to be present, it should only be with the informed consent of the woman. The staff who are present will include technical, midwifery/nursing, anaesthetic and obstetric/paediatric person-nel. The number of neonatal staff will vary according to the number of babies being born.

The person who is also almost certain to be present is the woman's partner or chosen birth companion. The father's entrance into the birthing room in the late twentieth century was followed surprisingly quickly by his admission into the caesarean theatre (Mander, 2004a). The reason for this being surprising relates to the general perception of the father's role in the birthing room. He was considered to be there to help and support his partner in her labour. It is difficult to imagine how this could apply in the operating theatre, yet he was, albeit grudgingly, accepted. This acceptance, though, is less than complete. For many of the fathers, if his partner is given a general anaesthetic, he is excluded.

The rationale for this apparently irrational veto on the father's presence is explained by staff on the ARM website (2001):

> A C/Section is a major operation, one of the many risks is that of infection, so ideally a minimum number of people should be in theatre. The idea of having someone with you for the C/S is for support for you . . . a birth partner. If you are asleep, then that person has no need to be there. (Janet, 2001)

> The reason given at our unit is that the birth partner is there to do just that give support and if the woman has a GA then she is asleep and there is no need for him/her to be in theatre. They can go with them to the door and we bring them into recovery afterwards. (Donna, 2001)

The women's disappointment, though, is clear in their comments:

> My husband was banned from theatre, resulting in my son's birth being a total mystery to the both of us. (Emma, 2001)

> neither I nor my husband witnessed our birth. (Angela C., 2001)

One woman recounts her partner's anxiety:

> My husband describes very clearly his feelings of being left totally alone in a corridor for 20 minutes, not knowing if either of us were alive or dead . . . to be left alone with no support or information and neither parent 'present' at the birth is no way to start family life. (Jenny, 2001)

The significance of this problem is analysed by one woman and conclusions drawn:

> For some couples, being present is even more important when the woman is under GA because they feel strongly that the father at least should be present to welcome their baby into the world. It should boil down to the couple being given the full facts about what to expect so that they make an informed decision about whether it is appropriate for them to be present or not. I would suggest that refusal to 'allow' the father to be present is just yet another example of patriarchy in action. (Lorna, 2001)

The father's serious misgivings about this experience emerged serendipitously in a small study in Heidelberg, Germany (Koppel and Kaiser, 2001). These researchers planned a qualitative study to examine the experience of the father with a baby in the neonatal intensive care unit (NICU). A sample of 18 fathers of newborn babies was recruited. The fathers were keen to talk to the researcher but, unfortunately for the research design, not to talk about their experience of being the father of a baby in an NICU.

The fathers' major concern hinged on the birth of the baby, which for most of the informants was by caesarean under general anaesthesia. Of the 18 births, 17 were by caesarean. Four of these fathers were present at the birth. Of the remaining 13, 10 (77 per cent) of the fathers were shocked to find that they were prevented from being with their partner during the birth. The reason given to these men for their exclusion was that the caesarean was being performed under a general anaesthetic. These fathers were excluded in spite of 'heated debates and/or desperate pleas' (2001:250). Thus, the situation arises of the father ordinarily being encouraged to accompany his partner at the birth, but, when his presence would later be most helpful, his presence is effectively vetoed. The paradoxical nature of this scenario has been noted previously by Oakley and Richards (1990).

The researchers focus on the fathers' emotional reactions to their exclusion, hence the highly graphic title of the paper 'Fathers at the end of their rope'. This title is a more emotive translation of the rather British 'end of their tether'. The apparent change in the direction of the rope from horizontal to vertical carries sinister allusions. As well as the fathers being unsurprisingly distraught, they complained vehemently about the lack of information. For this reason their disenchantment was aggravated by their anxiety about their partner and their baby. Thus, the unanswered question remains: What is the father's role that he is able to perform at a caesarean with regional anaesthesia that he can't perform when a general anaesthetic is used?

In addition to the research by Koppel and Kaiser (2001), Clement's study (1995) shows the emotional sequelae of the father's exclusion. One father, having psyched himself up to attend the birth, reported that he felt 'discarded as no one at the last minute. I was robbed' (1995:139). The woman might, as a result, later feel guilty on her partner's behalf. Such misgivings could all too easily damage the fledgling family relationships. Such damage appears to be particularly likely if and when the father 'meets' the baby while the woman is still asleep: 'I felt that my husband and son formed part of a family from which I was excluded and I was terribly jealous of them and their relationship' (1995:140).

3.4 Conclusion

In this chapter I have sought to address the technical, surgery-related issues which may have shorter- or longer-term repercussions for the childbearing woman. While the intention was originally to provide merely the technical background for the more important aspects which feature in other parts of this book, what has emerged is different. This largely technical material has proved in itself to matter to the experience of the childbearing woman undergoing a caesarean. Thus, particularly for those providing care, it is necessary to bear in mind that no aspect is too trivial or too technical for it to carry huge significance for the woman experiencing it.

4 International matters

The links between technological and other developments in the wealthier countries and what happens in the low- and middle-income countries may not always be obvious. The nature of the interrelationship in the context of perinatal health care is due to globalisation.

(Chalmers, 2004:890)

4.1 International background

In spite of Chalmers's characteristically profound observation, 'globalisation' is becoming something of a cliché. Its decline is aggravated by it being a word which is frequently, and frequently wrongly, used. So globalisation deserves explaining. Rather than meaning an internationalist approach or regionalisation, it refers to those processes which convert the world into one single entity. This in itself may be no bad thing, but when we remember that these processes lead to the removal of national, cultural and linguistic boundaries, globalisation's potentially dire implications become clear (Bettcher and Lee, 2002).

In the context of health care provision, as well as in other 'industries', these implications have been foretold. A major instrument of globalisation has been the World Trade Organisation (WTO) which, in conjunction with transnational corporations (TNCs) has brought about the eradication of public funding streams (Pollock and Price, 2000). In health care, the demise of public funding has led to the abolition of many services and the introduction of funding systems such as PFI (private finance initiative) and PPP (public private partnership).

The increasing influence of international agencies like the WTO, which supposedly regulates world trade, and the World Bank is disconcerting (Walt, 1998). Not only does the power of international organisations threaten the welfare of the low- and middle-income countries, it also jeopardises the functioning of other more specialised agencies such as the World Health Organisation.

4.1.1 The role of the World Health Organisation (WHO)

Although the credentials of the World Health Organisation are relatively unblemished, its record in the context of reproductive health may leave something to be desired. Using the woman's experience as the starting point, the WHO partograph (see section 3.1.1), which may also be known as the partogram, merits attention first.

The partograph originated as a 'cervicograph' in Zimbabwe (Philpott, 1972) to simply record the woman's progress in labour by graphically illustrating cervical dilatation. To the 'progress' line was later added an 'alert' line and an 'action' line. These were intended to indicate the need for transfer to a higher level of health care and augmentation of labour (see Figure 4.1). The aim was to avoid prolonged labour by intervening with the timely use of oxytocic drugs. The research basis of the introduction of the partograph has been shown to be gravely defective (Lavender, 2003).

Any systematic evaluation was delayed until 1994 when a study of the effects of using the World Health Organisation partograph was undertaken in South East Asia (WHO, 1994). As with the introduction of the original document, this partograph's evaluation was also 'deeply flawed' (Rosser, 1994). The omission of a randomised controlled trial and the introduction of a 'package' of confounding interventions render the 1994 evaluation seriously faulty. A further evaluation of the partograph was undertaken later, to assess the effects on women's satisfaction of differing time periods between the alert and the action lines (Lavender et al, 1999).

While Lavender and her colleagues recognise the association between partograph use and caesarean rates, this was not the focus of their study. It is necessary to consider the nature of the association between the routine intervention, which is the use of the partograph, and caesarean. The connection is found in the requirement that if the woman's progress line falls below the action line on the partograph, then action becomes mandatory. This interventive action involves the augmentation or acceleration of the woman's labour by rupturing the membranes and/or administering an oxytocic drug. Thus, the potential exists for the establishment of the cascade of intervention which may, ultimately, lead to a caesarean (see section 3.3.1). This potential danger in the use of the partograph has been observed and reported in an Australian context. It was found there to 'lead to increased action, rather than assessment' (Groeschel and Glover, 2001:26).

The second blemish on the WHO reproductive health record is even more directly relevant to the caesarean operation. This blemish happened at a meeting in Fortaleza, Brazil attended by midwives, obstetricians, paediatricians, epidemiologists, sociologists, psychologists, health administrators and mothers (Lancet, 1985). The meeting, according to Beech (2004), was called by WHO in an attempt to address the persistently and globally increasing rates of medicalisation of childbirth. The participants undertook a painstaking review of the research evidence, on the basis of which a number of recommendations were prepared. The recommendations, which covered a wide range of areas, addressed general and specific issues as well as their implementation. The recommendations were preceded by a slightly

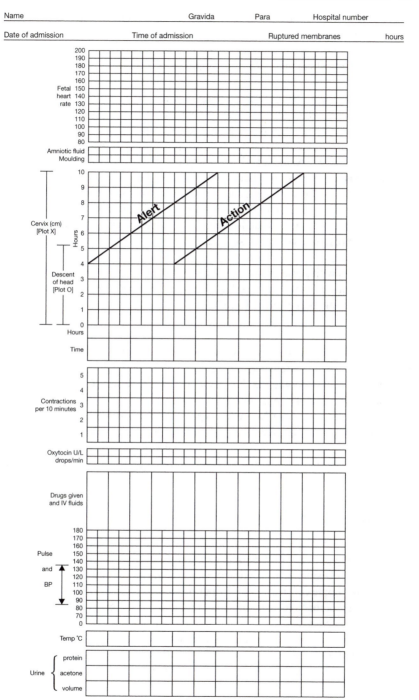

Figure 4.1 The WHO Partograph.

disconcerting 'disclaimer' to the effect that: 'even "no risk pregnancies" can give rise to complications. Sometimes intervention is required to obtain the best result' (Lancet, 1985:436). While such statements may be technically accurate, they reflect a disturbingly medical view of healthy childbearing.

Beech reports that she was 'the lay representative for the whole of Europe' (2004:1). She recounts how the meeting reached its most notable or notorious recommendation, which related to the optimal caesarean rate. There was agreement among the participants that the evidence indicated that there is no justification for a caesarean rate greater than 10 per cent. In spite of this decision being otherwise unanimous, the two American obstetric representatives 'threw up their hands in horror' (2004:1). They argued that were such a low rate to be recommended, other obstetricians would regard the recommendations as nothing more than a joke and ignore them. As so often happens when a small but powerful group threatens to jeopardise a resolution, a mutually acceptable concession was negotiated. On this occasion the resulting compromise reads:

> Countries with some of the lowest perinatal mortality rates in the world have caesarean section rates of less than 10%. There is no justification for any region to have a rate higher than 10–15%.
>
> (Lancet, 1985: 437)

Beech records her 'disquiet' at what is clearly a flagrant reduction of the impact, which, she correctly anticipated, would lead to the lower figure being ignored and 15 per cent would become the 'ball park' figure. Of course, Cassandra-like, she has had the dubious pleasure of being proved right.

Thus, in these two caesarean-related examples, the World Health Organisation has failed abysmally to cover itself with glory. It might even be suggested that, although this organisation is charged with safeguarding world *health*, its mission appears to be to maintain world *medicalisation*, at least in the context of child-bearing.

4.1.2 Accuracy of caesarean rates

Much of the concern about caesareans relates to the increase in the rate or the numbers being performed. It is usual to assume that such statistics are factual and that Benjamin Disraeli's accusation of 'Lies, damned lies and statistics' does not apply in this context. There is a distinct possibility, however, that data may be unreliable and/or incomplete in low-income countries (Hyder and Morrow, 2001:5). This is associated with even the collection of vital statistics relating to births and deaths being only partial. By way of illustration, Hyder and Morrow report that in 1990 only two out of eight regions of the world were able to claim the complete registration of vital statistics. It may be that, in comparison, recording the *mode* or *route* of birth becomes a very low priority. Part of the reason for inaccuracies may be found in the variations in the training and expertise of the staff handling the data. These variations may be aggravated by unsatisfactory supervision and limited feedback. Hyder and Morrow express confidence, though, in the likelihood that the situation is getting better.

In connection with specifically childbearing-related statistics, incomplete reporting may be due to value judgements concerning the pregnancy being reported (Menken and Rahman, 2001:118). If a health condition does not reflect well on the society in which it occurs, attempts may be made to disguise its existence. Caesarean is an example of such a condition, reflecting as it does the woman's failure to complete 'that most-valued achievement of a successful pregnancy – a spontaneous delivery at home' (Kwast, 1996:5). In the case of a condition which cannot be disguised, such as a maternal death, the cause may be attributed to a more socially 'acceptable' condition. This may result in the figures for more acceptable conditions, such as haemorrhage, being artificially inflated, compared with, for example, infection.

The difficulties of collecting reliable data, particularly in low-income countries, are clearly apparent and the reasons are probably understandable. The extent to which any of these difficulties apply in higher-income countries is open to conjecture.

4.1.3 Significance of caesarean rates

While the rates are globally significant, the reason for the significance of the rates varies according to the context. In developing countries the caesarean rate may be used as an indication of the quality of maternity care in, for example, the Safe Motherhood Programme (Stanton et al, 2005). These authors caution, though, that the rate may be inflated by the caesarean decision increasingly being based on fetal rather than maternal indications. They go on to assert that, even in developing countries where resources are at a premium, a high caesarean rate may conceal a large number of quite unnecessary operations. This situation may even apply in settings where there may simultaneously be an unmet need for life-saving caesareans. In this way the already appalling maternal mortality rates are further aggravated by the lack of appropriate caesarean operations. It is apparent that a serious imbalance between need and provision has been identified in some areas.

4.1.4 Health systems

Because of the influence of the organisation of health care on that care, it is necessary to consider the ways in which differing health care systems are associated with varying caesarean rates. Having suggested the link between health systems and care, though, we should not lose sight of the indissoluble link between those systems and the communities of people from which they arise and whom they exist to serve. In this way, I suggest that the local culture may be, to some extent, reflected in health care. Of course, a range of other factors also exert an influence, including history, climate and geography (Sharpe and Faden, 1998).

In considering the implications of health systems for an intervention such as caesarean, it is crucial to bear in mind their dynamic nature. As I have observed elsewhere, health systems 'have a tendency not to remain the same for very long' (Mander, 2001a:21). While this observation was made in the context of wealthy western countries, it may be that it applies equally to middle- and low-income states. This dynamism of health systems may be due in part to the process of globalisation mentioned already. Another, not totally unconnected, factor is the political nature of health care, which reflects both its funding and its provision.

The balance of power within the health system is largely determined by the extent of its market orientation. In a publicly funded system, there may be a tension between the bureaucracy or the possibly democratically elected policy-makers and the providers of care. The latter occupational or professional groups may themselves constitute a political entity, but they have a tendency to reinforce the regulatory power exercised by the state (Johnson, 1995).

In those states where health care is provided according to a 'free market' system, competition and consumer choice are held to feature prominently. The effectiveness and availability of these features, respectively, may owe more to rhetoric than to reality, though. The accessibility and equity of the health care system refers not only to the services provided and geography and transport, but additionally to a range of cultural and social phenomena which will be addressed in the next section. Closely linked to both accessibility and funding arrangements is the method of payment. Although even publicly funded health systems, which derive their income from taxation or insurance payments, rely to some extent on out of pocket payments by patients or clients and their relatives (Levitt et al, 1995:270).

4.1.5 Sociocultural factors

The way in which social, cultural and economic aspects of peoples' lives impact on their health is becoming increasingly clear. This impact is visited particularly on women (Doyal, 2001), even in the most affluent countries. In the low-income countries, however, the woman's position is worse than in wealthier ones because of a generally lower standard of living and smaller health budget. The annual per capita expenditure on health care is $5,274 in the USA at the time of writing (WHO, 2006); in Nepal, however, the figure is $6.4. Women are particularly disadvantaged in such circumstances because their social standing may be lower than their men folk, as is their contribution to decision making. So, even if the woman is able to decide that health care is needed, she does not have access to the financial resources to pay for the journey. The woman's difficulty is further aggravated by women's tendency to prioritise their children's spending needs over their own.

If the woman is in a setting where her 'honour' needs to be 'guarded' by her men folk, she may be forbidden from travelling unaccompanied. Further, if there were a risk that the health care provider would be male, any contact would be prohibited. The woman's crucial role as a source of unpaid labour may mean that she is, effectively, indispensable. Women's stereotypical low self-esteem may further aggravate the problems they experience in accessing health care (WHO, 1998).

The nature of the health care available to women may also limit her choices. A glance at the literature shows that the priorities of a range of aid organisations are, probably appropriately, on the prevention of unwanted pregnancy and ensuring the health of young children. Such priorities mean that there is little left over for women's health.

In the field of childbearing there exists the potential for strongly held cultural beliefs to conflict with the views of health care providers. This danger is most likely if a western medical model of health is being applied in a setting where it is antithetical to the local ethos. It may be necessary to bear in mind, though, that the reverse may be the case. In such a situation, medicalised, high-tech, 'western' health care may be perceived as better and more effective. Thus, it will be higher status than more basic or traditional approaches. For these reasons, western health care is likely to be widely sought after.

4.2 Comparisons between countries

Much of the concern about increasing numbers of caesareans is associated with the variations in the rates between countries which may otherwise be comparable. I consider here the caesarean situation in a number of areas/countries in ascending order of their wealth, as indicated by their gross domestic product (GDP) (WHO, 2006). In examining these rates, I draw attention to the multiplicity of issues which have been shown to influence caesarean rates.

4.2.1 Low-income states

In a general overview of the problems associated with caesarean in 'developing countries' (Kwawukume, 2001:165), the reader is reminded of the conditions in which so many women give birth. These conditions are fundamentally different from those to which westerners have become accustomed. Shortages are prevalent, such as lack of transport, communication and other resources, eg staff, blood products and basic services. Although women are prepared to attend for antenatal care, they may be reluctant to seek admission to a maternity unit because of its association with assisted or operative outcomes. Such interventions are not favoured because spontaneous birth is traditionally so highly desirable as a natural function. Assistance or surgery are deprecated because they demonstrate the woman's inability to complete this function. Caesarean may be additionally unpopular because women who would like a large family believe that caesarean may limit their fertility (Kwawukume, 2001). Indeed in one particular setting this fear is justified. This involved the surgeon briefly applying Spencer Wells forceps to the woman's fallopian tubes during the early stage of the suturing. The rationale was that, by so doing, a future pregnancy, a ruptured uterus and a maternal death was being prevented. Clearly, in ethical terms, such an action is totally reprehensible.

If a woman in labour is thought to need admission, her husband may need to give his consent. Because of the distances involved, the labouring woman may then have to travel a long way either on foot or in uncongenial transport over difficult terrain to reach maternity care. Prolonged or obstructed labour may be present prior to such a journey or may supervene. Obstructed labour is not uncommonly associated with cephalo-pelvic disproportion (CPD) in low-income countries, often being due to malformation of the pelvic bones through childhood disease.

While a major degree of CPD carries mortality risks for the woman and baby, a lesser degree carries with it the risk of a more insidious and longer-term form of morbidity. This is the formation of a fistula. Because of pressure of the baby's head on the bony pelvis during a prolonged or obstructed labour, the woman's anterior and posterior tissues are effectively crushed, leading to tissue death or necrosis. Following the birth the healing of these necrotic areas causes a channel to form between the structures that were crushed. Thus, a vesico-vaginal fistula may form between the bladder and the vagina, and/or a recto-vaginal fistula may form between the rectum and the vagina. The formation of a fistula means that the woman becomes incontinent of urine and/or faeces, respectively.

Figures are not easily available for the incidence of fistula formation, but it is a significant cause of maternal morbidity in low- and middle-income countries (Menken and Rahman, 2001:120). The woman's incontinence renders her socially and sexually unacceptable. She is likely to be abandoned by her husband, stigmatised by society and ostracised. Her unclean status will prevent her from being involved in that most womanly function of food preparation. Being considered 'polluted' and 'polluting' will mean that she will be excluded from religious observance. While fistula is not actually a cause of maternal mortality, it might certainly be considered to be a cause of a slow and lingering 'social death'. The part which men play in the development and effects of these conditions needs to be recognised. It is now being proposed that men should be better educated about women's health issues in order to reduce their frequency and impact (Kwawukume, 2001). Part of this educational function is being undertaken by organisations such as 'O Renew' (UNPF, 2006).

Thus, I am advancing the argument that the lack of resources in low-income states, together with some societal factors, means that access is lacking to necessary caesarean operations. In further support of this, Buekens and colleagues (2003) analyse data on eight sub-Saharan countries. They suggest that in this region an appropriate caesarean rate to address maternal complications would be about 5.4 per cent. These researchers' data show that caesarean rates are generally rising to come nearer the optimal rate. Kenya, though, is the only country with a rate approaching that which is recommended. Clearly there is a need for women to have better access to caesarean in this area. At the same time, aid agencies must be careful to avoid stimulating an increase in the number of *unnecessary* caesareans which would cause 'iatrogenic mortality and morbidity' (2003:136). Thus, caesareans need to be employed appropriately, rather than as currently being over-used in some settings and unobtainable in others.

In a study of caesarean use in Kerala, India, some traditional beliefs, such as astrology, were found to influence its use (Padmadas et al, 2000). In this area, which is relatively well provided with health care facilities, these researchers found a significant difference between practice in the public and the private hospitals. They show that the caesarean rate is 1.7 times higher when the woman attends an obstetrician privately. This finding clearly endorses Buekens and colleagues' concerns about the inappropriate use of caesarean in lower-income countries.

In Jordan, a six-year collection of data clearly demonstrates the inexorable rise, to the point of doubling, of the caesarean rate in one maternity unit (Akasheh and Amarin, 2000). Whereas caesarean may often be justified on the grounds that it avoids a hazardous assisted birth using forceps, in this situation the forceps rate was unaffected by the increase in caesareans. The number of assisted births using vacuum extraction, though, appears to have fallen reciprocally. Akasheh and Amarin discuss 'physician-related' indications for caesarean (2000:44), by which they mean obstetricians' misguided adherence to the old adage 'once a caesarean, always a caesarean' (see section 8.1.1). Fatalistically, though, they argue that this attitude is not amenable to change; rather, that the number of primary caesareans must be reduced if the 'caesarean epidemic' is to be brought under control.

4.2.2 China

In terms of its gross domestic product, China is more or less on a par with Jordan. China's phenomenal rate of development together with its astounding contrasts, though, mean that it merits special attention. At the time of writing, China is in the throes of converting itself into a twenty-first-century socialist-capitalist state with a free market economy (Casetti, 2003). In spite of these developments, China's human rights and democratic credentials are woefully inadequate. One of the human rights abuses, the one child policy, which was introduced in 1980 and became law in 1982 (Cheung, 2006), has been influential in the accelerating rate of caesarean there. Cultural factors have also contributed. These include the relatively high esteem in which medical practitioners and their interventions are held. Another factor is the traditionally low status of the woman in relation to her mother-in-law until the woman gives birth to a son (Cheung, 2000).

A further problem is the position of the midwife in China (Cheung et al, 2005a). This is associated with the medical model of childbearing which was imported from the USA, together with a wide range of other changes in culture. The result for maternity care is not dissimilar to what was happening about a century earlier in the USA (Jackson and Mander, 1995). By this I mean that in 1993 midwifery was deemed non-essential and so midwifery education was discontinued. The midwives, who trained before 1993, have become nurses or medical practitioners, or possibly 'doulas' since 1996. It is the nursing staff in the labour wards who have now assumed the title of 'midwives' (Cheung et al, 2005a).

The demise of midwives and midwifery happened at the same time as more and more medical practitioners were being educated, which has been happening since 1972. Because of their traditionally higher status, a widespread assumption that they offer safer care, their unwillingness to work in the rural areas and their greater numbers, medical practitioners took over many midwifery functions relating to healthy childbirth. Thus, the medicalisation of childbirth escalated exponentially.

The extent of this medicalisation means that the caesarean rate has reached 100 per cent in some Chinese maternity units (Cheung et al, 2006).

It may be said, therefore, that this phenomenal caesarean rate is associated with changes in maternity and obstetric practice, which have been fuelled by cultural developments. Although the research by Cheung and colleagues suggests that Chinese women have wholeheartedly welcomed many of the cultural changes in the field of childbearing, it is necessary to recall that these changes originated with a policy imposed by a less than democratic regime.

4.2.3 The Latin American States and Brazil

The extraordinarily high rates of caesarean in Latin America in general and Brazil in particular have quite appropriately attracted considerable media attention. In the private hospitals there, the rates reach levels as high as 98 per cent (Nuttall, 2000) or 99 per cent (McCallum, 2005). In their research, Belizán and colleagues (1999) analysed the caesarean rates in 19 of the Latin American countries. This 'ecological study' compared the characteristics of populations, rather than the usual focus on the characteristics of individuals in case/control, cohort and randomised control trial designs.

As has been mentioned above (section 4.1.2), these researchers identify the challenges which they encountered in collecting data in countries whose priority is not the accumulation of statistics. In Latin America a positive correlation was identified between the caesarean rate and the standard of living, which was assessed in this study by the gross national product (GNP). While the collection of these data must be recognised as no mean feat, it is unfortunate that so little attention was given to the place of birth and attendant involved in vaginal births. The environment and the personnel involved may yet be shown to be of significance.

In Brazil, Béhague and colleagues (2002, see section 2.4.1) sought to probe the well-worn yet still thorny question of who is responsible for the increasing caesarean rates. A combination of both epidemiological and ethnographic methods were used to investigate whether medical intervention or women's demands were to blame. Although the word is not actually used, it appears that the culture of the country in general and maternity in particular must be held responsible. Especially important is the interaction between the childbearing woman and her medical attendant. The researchers exemplify situations where a shared background and common values lead to a birth which satisfies both groups, in the form of a caesarean. For women who do not share that background or those values, though, the situation is very different. Thus, for women who are young, unmarried, poor or any combination of these, an antagonism arises which leads to traumatic birthing experiences:

> Maria: The doctor felt nauseous when he looked at me because I didn't do antenatal care, they don't like people who don't do antenatal care.
>
> (Béhague et al, 2002:944)

Andrezza: I told him, 'Oh, Mr doctor, you don't have the guts that I do!' Then I tried kicking him, but the lady doctor told me to calm down, to not act like that, because otherwise they would mistreat me . . .

(Béhague et al, 2002:944)

It may not be surprising that in such circumstances women endeavour to avoid such confrontations in labour by seeking birth by caesarean, a finding endorsed by Potter and colleagues (2001). It may be suggested that the problem in such a situation lies not in the birth intervention, but in the maternity system. For these reasons, these researchers make the disconcerting observation that 'those with greatest need for caesarean sections were the least likely to receive one' (Béhague et al, 2002:943).

The culture in Brazil is further addressed in terms of the status of caesarean. This operation is high status, in comparison to nurse-midwives, whose status is so low as to prevent them from finding employment (Nuttall, 2000). Such a situation is aggravated by the perception that, for obstetricians, 'time is money', and they are unable to wait for a spontaneous or other vaginal birth. Because of their system of education, medical students' surgical skills are prioritised over their 'midwifery skills' (McCallum, 2005:231). The result is that practitioners opt for what they are best able to do, surgical births, rather than risk litigation.

Of special interest in Nuttall's cultural analysis is her observation of the influence of religion in inflating the Brazilian caesarean rate (2000). She identifies the paradoxical attitude found in Roman Catholic countries towards women's bodies. Whereas the woman's role as a mother is a source of reverence, the man's attitude to the woman's body is that it is there solely for his sexual gratification, rather than for giving birth to children. It appears that Brazilian women may be subjugated to their men folk, particularly through the childbearing cycle from conception to birth. It has been argued that such subjugation, including caesarean, may constitute another form of violence against women (Castro, 1999).

4.2.4 Greece

The Greek health care system has undergone three major reforms since the introduction of care free at the point of receipt in 1983. Such a high number of corrective measures are an indication of the severity of the challenges facing this fledgling health service. Nikolentzos demonstrates some of the reasons by contrasting the weakness of the Greek state with the power of the major 'actors' in the health care system (2005:2). These actors comprise the trade unions, the health insurance funds and, of course, the medical profession. This maelstrom of vested interests provides the backdrop to the experience of the childbearing woman and the likelihood of her undergoing a caesarean. These interest groups and the relationships between them were explored by examining the caesarean rates in three Greek hospitals (Mossialos et al, 2005). The considerable involvement of insurance companies is demonstrated by the massive private component of the health system, which at 44 per cent is the greatest proportion in the European Union (EU). This study identified caesarean rates of 41.6 per cent in the public and 53 per cent in the private institutions.

As well as the funding situation, the medical profession is also in a predicament due to the serious oversupply of medical practitioners. The problem is that Greece has the highest ratio of specialist physicians to population in the EU and the total number of medical practitioners has doubled in the past two decades (Nikolentzos, 2005). On the other hand, the number of registered nurses is approximately half the EU average. The quality of the Greek nursing profession has been seriously diluted by the employment of assistant nurses during times of shortage; subsequently, these unqualified staff are unable to be dislodged from their posts (Plati et al, 1998). The result is that, although there is now a steady supply of registered nurses, there are no posts available for them. Thus, for a number of reasons, it would appear that the power balance in Greek health care is weighted very much in favour of the medical fraternity.

The relationship between this vast army of under-employed medical practitioners and the insurance companies is interesting and may be summarised as 'cosy' (Mossialos et al, 2005). This results in what has, elsewhere, been termed 'insurance-led care' (Mander, 1997). Mossialos and his colleagues, though, refer to this phenomenon as 'supplier-induced demand for [caesarean]' (2005:293). They go on to outline how the 'commercialization' of maternity care in Greece (2005:295) has exacerbated its difficulties. This process has included the floating of private hospitals on the stock market in the late 1990s. Further, high 'informal payments' to obstetricians for performing caesareans (2005:295) cannot but have influenced their clinical decision making. The cultural phenomenon which is known as '*Fakellaki*', or backhanders, operates at many levels throughout Greek society and there is probably no reason why health care should be immune (Kasidi, 2006). Thus, Greek obstetricians are clearly motivated to perform caesareans by the availability of 'financial and convenience incentives' (Mossialos et al, 2005:295).

The powerful position of the obstetrician in Greece may be a reflection of the weak position of the midwife. My reading and a search of CINAHL and the web for the words 'Greek midwife' or 'Greek midwifery' produced only references to the ancients. Whether a midwifery profession which is so low profile as to be invisible is beneficial to the childbearing woman is an issue which needs to be addressed.

4.2.5 Israel

The ongoing conflicts between Israel and its neighbours clearly carry a multitude of issues for the members of the embattled communities. While many difficulties may be overcome by local negotiation (Cohen, 2005), others exert serious challenges to individuals and to agencies such as the health care and maternity services. Of particular significance is the difficulty of travelling due to the multitude of armed roadblocks and military checkpoints. Thus, antenatal care and care during labour and birth may be unpredictable. While Jewish families are able to access seriously medicalised health care (Filc, 2005), Palestinian women are more likely to suffer the indignity and trauma of giving birth in an ambulance held up at an army check-point. Because of the imposition of travel restrictions since the second *intifada*, young women's educational opportunities have been seriously curtailed. Due in part to these two phenomena, girls and young women often marry within their extended family at the relatively early age of fifteen. The implications of this arrangement for perinatal health have yet to be fully assessed.

In spite of these difficulties in some locations, a nurse-midwife practising in a university hospital has been able to establish her woman-centred credentials (Slome, 2002). In the same setting, though, there are concerns that the caesarean rate in Israel doubled to 18 per cent between 1984 and 2003 (Cohain and Yoselis, 2004). These researchers retrospectively compared one unit's caesarean rates among 'low-risk' women who gave birth in 1990 with those who gave birth in 2000. The definition of what is meant by 'low-risk' is always problematical, but Cohain and Yoselis assessed risk using a well-validated instrument. The maternity unit serves a relatively homogeneous and affluent population and there are about 4,800 births per annum. The researchers identified a significant increase in the caesarean rate from 4 per cent to 10.5 per cent. This increase comprised a doubling of the emergency caesarean rate from 3.2 per cent to 6.7 per cent, but the elective caesarean rate quintupled from 0.7 per cent to 3.7 per cent. The conclusion is drawn that such increases 'must be due to non-medical factors' and the researchers blame practice which is not evidence-based, defensive obstetrics or 'time of day' (2004:31).

While this latter reason sounds slightly odd, many who are acquainted with obstetrics will recognise the tendency to choose to undertake an 'emergency' caesarean 'when staff are available', rather than at less sociable hours. This obser-vation is supported by finding that there is a significant increase in the number of 'emergency' caesareans between 08.00 and 14.00 (Goldstick et al, 2003). In comparison, the proportion undertaken between 05.00 and 06.00 is minuscule. This tendency is attributed to the 'convenience' of the operator being a major factor in deciding not only to actually undertake an emergency caesarean, but also *when* it should be undertaken (Cohain and Yoselis, 2004).

Thus, the implications of civil strife for the childbearing woman are all too easily apparent. While one group of women are being forced to give birth in the back of an ambulance, the other group is undergoing emergency caesareans at the convenience of the obstetrician.

4.2.6 Australia

The traditionally significantly over-medicalised Australian maternity health care system is reported as beginning to experience some changes in the direction of a more midwife-led system (EGAMS, 2003). This process, however, is far from straightforward and even less complete (Robertson, 2004). In fact, Walker and colleagues appear to revel in their boast of, at 23.3 per cent, having 'among the highest proportion of births by caesarean in the western world' (2004:117). A sig-nificant feature of the Australian health system is the large proportion of consumers who purchase private medical insurance. The number is as high as one third (Roberts et al, 2000), to which must be added those who choose to pay directly for private obstetric services. These researchers clearly demonstrate, as has been shown in other countries, the pointlessly high intervention and caesarean rates among women giving birth in private hospitals and who choose to 'go private' in public hospitals. Roberts and colleagues show the doubling of certain interventions among 'private patients' (2000:139), including elective caesarean, epidural and episiotomy. The interpretation of Roberts and colleagues' data (2002) is impeded by linguistic difficulties, such as using the term 'operative' to include not only caesarean operations, but also assisted vaginal births. Unlike the findings of Akasheh and Amarin (2000, please see section 4.2.1), the number of births assisted by vacuum extraction have increased approximately threefold, whereas the caesarean rate has increased by about 25 per cent.

The inability, though, of the 'caesarean section industry' to offer a panacea to childbearing women in Australia is argued by King (2000:125). In response to this argument, Walker and her colleagues sought to investigate the part played by cultural beliefs in the 'excessive use of caesarean' (2004:117). These researchers suggest that one factor may be the woman's 'loyalty' to her birth experience (2004:118). This is taken to mean the woman's tendency to persuade herself that her method of birth was 'right' and hence reassure herself that, irrespective of the route of birth, it was the best one for her and her baby. Walker and colleagues used a Likert-type scale to access women's perceptions of the community acceptance of caesarean. This data collection technique shows the respondent a, usually, five-point scale on which to agree or disagree with statements relating to the topic. In order to persuade the respondent to engage thoughtfully with the topic, it is usual to use a mixture of positive and negative statements, which are then coded and scored appropriately resulting in a positive/negative weighting. In Walker and colleagues' instrument, though, the statements are not balanced in this way, but all are positive towards caesarean:

'CS is no longer seen as major surgery'
'CS is now seen as a routine way of having a baby'
'It is common for people to think that CS offers an easier way of giving birth'

(Walker et al, 2004:121).

In view of these overwhelmingly positive statements, it may have been more difficult for women to disagree with them. Thus, the sample of new mothers generally agreed that caesarean is perceived as being easy and convenient. This criticism, though, does not question the immense changes in public perceptions about the advantages of caesarean. The Australian moves towards midwife-led care (Homer et al, 2002) appear to be happening in spite of such cultural impediments. The role of the midwife in that country still appears to be comparatively marginal, judging from their absence from the caesarean literature and the perceived need for obstetricians to 'supervise' women in labour (King, 2000:125).

4.2.7 The Netherlands

The Dutch system of maternity care is world famous. It functions within a health service which provides a public system of care for people whose income is below a certain level, and a private scheme for those with a higher income (EGAMS, 2003). In this small country of just over sixteen million people, access to services is easy in terms of both physical proximity and organisation (Mander, 1995b). Another important factor in the success of the Dutch maternity services lies in the status of midwifery practice, which for historical reasons is seriously high (Marland, 1993). This is in marked contrast to many other countries where midwives are, at best, marginalised. In the Netherlands, the generally accepted assumption is that childbearing is a healthy process. This is evidenced by maternity care ordinarily being provided by a midwife. The assumption is that the childbearing woman does not necessarily need the attention of a medical practitioner. Medical care may be provided, though, if a midwife is not available or if complications arise (den Exter et al, 2004).

One outcome of this system is that approximately one third of births in the Netherlands happen in the woman's home. Another result is that the caesarean rate is probably the lowest for a western country at the end of the twentieth century, at 11.2 per cent (Declercq and Viisainen, 2001). In this small state, the usual rule of a correlation between high socio-economic status and higher caesarean rates appears to have been broken. This features in the research on 'elderly nulliparae' which found that, although there were more referrals in labour among the older and more affluent group, the caesarean rate was not significantly raised (Smit et al, 1997).

This exceptional finding is further illuminated by research into the relationship between the community income and surgical interventions in general (Westert et al, 2003). These researchers used the women's and men's 'community of residence' to estimate their income level. It emerged that those women whose income was highest were least likely to have a caesarean and that the equivalent men were equally unlikely to have surgery.

The success of the Dutch maternity system in keeping birth 'normal' is usually attributed to the local culture. I would venture to suggest that this 'normal' orientation is tied in with the strength and longstanding nature of the midwifery presence. The limited opportunities for private obstetric practice may be another important factor. It may be assumed that the importance of culture also applies to the use of the caesarean. The role of the Dutch midwife is widely recognised as crucial in maintaining 'normality'. Perhaps we may also assume that the midwife contributes to the other side of this 'coin', that is, to the low caesarean rates.

4.2.8 Ireland

The Republic of Ireland, with a population of about 3.5 million, suffered in the late twentieth century from a momentous depopulation crisis. This, together with the seriously falling birth rate observed in many formerly strict Roman Catholic states, is resulting in a shortage of health care personnel (EGAMS, 2003). The labourforce crisis clearly carries grave implications for maternity care and the use of caesarean. A survey in 1998 identified a national caesarean rate of 17.8 per cent, with a rate as high as 26.7 per cent in one centre (Farah et al, 2003). These researchers were disconcerted to find that the caesarean rate had tripled in the 16 years since 1982. Unlike the countries considered already, it has not been possible to locate details of the size of the private health care industry in Ireland, but there is only one private maternity unit, which is in Dublin (EGAMS, 2003).

The surprise among Farah and colleagues at the escalating caesarean rate may be due to the Irish figures having traditionally been more notable for their low level. Their notability, or perhaps notoriety, derives from the work of O'Driscoll and his colleagues (2003) at the National Maternity Hospital (Holles Street) in Dublin. These low caesarean rates have attracted admiring glances from North America, because of the spiralling rates and associated costs there (see section 4.2.9). These rates have been perceived to be a major spin off of the 'Dublin protocol', an interventive regime of medicalised care in labour. Research and emulation have followed and in the form of the entrée on to the childbearing stage of the 'doula' (Mander, 2001b). The success of the Dublin regime, according to the obstetricians, is dependent on continuous personal attention during labour, although this attendant is more likely to be a student than a qualified member of staff. This attendant is tasked with not only providing emotional support and completing clinical observations and care, but also maintaining constant eye contact. The obstetricians believe that the woman closing her eyes is of profound significance, indicating, it is maintained, a tendency to introspection, the onset of panic and 'the first step along the road to total disintegration' (O'Driscoll et al, 1993:93). The constant attention aims to prevent such deterioration; the availability of personnel to provide such care is facilitated by the unit policy of active, some would say aggressive, management of labour.

Thus, the Dublin regime presents a picture of a form of management of labour which verges on the 'military efficiency' to which the authors have referred (O'Driscoll and Meagher, 1986:89). It is this very efficiency which, we are told, facilitates the much admired system of support. The environment of care, though, is characterised by the dominance of the partograph to determine the timing and extent of interventions to accelerate labour. This labour environment has been appropriately described as 'neo-Taylorist' after 'FW Speedy Taylor', who was one of the early twentieth century's less humane occupational psychologists (Mason, 2000:247). It is necessary to consider whether the labour ward environment in Dublin's National Maternity Hospital is only rendered tolerable (if it is) by the constant companionship of the support person.

The question which I have not addressed yet, though, is how this regime relates to the famously low caesarean rates for first time mothers. An answer may be found in the data, which indicate the stage of labour at which women are admitted to the National Maternity Hospital (O'Driscoll et al, 1993:207). It should be noted that, in my experience, it is not usual for a maternity unit to record these figures. These data show that 5 per cent of first time mothers have achieved full dilatation of the cervix prior to admission to the maternity unit. In over 30 years as a midwife, though, I am unable to recall such a situation in uncomplicated childbirth. Thus, it is necessary to question whether the low rates of caesarean are due to this phenomenon, rather than to the support proffered by an unqualified person during labour. This question leads, in turn, to another about why the full dilatation on admission rate is so high among first time mothers? We may wonder whether there may, after all, be some truth to the infamous anecdote of labouring women sitting on a park bench opposite the National Maternity Hospital. In this way they are able, anecdotally, to delay as long as possible their admission and inevitable interventions and, coincidentally, avoid a caesarean.

4.2.9 *United States of America*

With a gross domestic product higher than any other country in the world, it should come as no surprise that health spending in the USA is also higher than any other country. To demonstrate the benefits of such spending it is useful to compare one particular aspect of health care with the situation in another country. Whereas in 2000 the USA spent an average of US$4178 on health care per head of the population, Poland spent only the equivalent of US$496 (Propper, 2001). In the same way, the USA spent 14 per cent of its GDP on health care whereas Poland, which was not far behind the UK, spent only 6 per cent of its GDP thus. These figures in themselves are relatively meaningless, until we come to look at the mortality rates in these two countries (OECD, 2005). I draw attention to the infant mortality rate (IMR) because, in the context of caesarean, it is a more appropriate indicator of a successful outcome than perinatal mortality. In 2003, in both of these hugely disparate countries the IMR was precisely the same at 7 per thousand live births. In terms of their IMR, these two countries were in the same 'ball park' as Hungary and Slovakia, with only Turkey and Mexico trailing some distance behind. I venture to suggest that it can only be a matter of time before the great American public realises the meaning of statistics such as these. The realisation will dawn that their health care system is not delivering health and that the extravagant costs are not being spent effectively. It is at this point that the health budget will cease to be just a sensitive issue, but will become a seriously political problem.

It is with this doomsday scenario in mind that any number of agencies are attempting to investigate and resolve the problem of the rising US caesarean rates. The rate of increase was, encouragingly, slowed by the arrival of the vaginal birth after caesarean (VBAC) movement in the early 1990s. This decline proved short-lived and by 2001 the figures had risen to exceed the 1990 level, with the increase at least as steep as previously (see Figure 4.2; Meikle et al, 2005). The national concern with these rates was sufficient to make reducing the caesarean rate a priority as one of the Healthy People Year 2000 objectives. An unsatisfactory evaluation shows, however, that this problem will still need to be included in the Year 2010 initiative.

One of the agencies seeking to address this problem is the National Center for Health Statistics (Menacker, 2005). The approach of this organisation is interesting

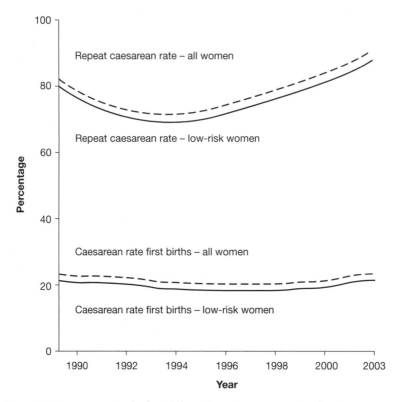

Figure 4.2 Caesarean rates for first births and repeat caesarean rates, for all women and low risk women in the USA, 1990–2003.

to the point of being novel. This agency, in presenting the caesarean statistics, separates out primary from secondary caesareans. Thus, a woman having her first (primary) caesarean is distinct from a woman having her second or subsequent (secondary) operation (Meikle et al, 2005). There may be more than one reason for this distinction. The first reason may relate to the presentation of the story. Figure 4.2 shows the differential between primary and secondary caesareans. The primary rate is considerably more acceptable, being lower, than the higher and more erratic secondary rate. This gives the impression that 'something is being done'. The second reason for this distinction, though, may be similarly devious. The secondary caesarean phenomenon may be considered to be part of an established culture of 'once a caesarean – always a caesarean' (see section 8.1). Culture is not easily amenable to change. The primary caesarean rate, though, reflects by definition a novel experience. It is this group of women who are the focus of the US onslaught. An attempt is being made to persuade first time mothers that their caesarean may not be really necessary. So, effectively, the higher and more significant secondary caesarean statistic is being written off as of no account, and the spotlight of attention is being turned on to the primary caesarean rate.

A not dissimilar strategy has been adopted to focus on an even smaller group who appear to, effectively, be being blamed for the rising caesarean rates (Meikle et al, 2005). These researchers criticise the terminology used to classify the indications for elective primary caesareans. Their wariness of the novel category 'abnormal fetal heart rate' on the grounds of imprecision (2005:754) is eminently reasonable. Their concern about increasing numbers of, for example, 'malpresentation' including breech presentation on grounds of an association with declining medical skills is probably appropriate. But to categorise the latter with 'maternal choice' ignores the crucial element of medical persuasion. Clearly, the concepts well recognised in creative accounting are being put to good use in 'creative statistics'. Thus, statisticians are being gainfully employed to assist with what appears to be becoming a new US national pastime of reducing, or possibly just massaging, the caesarean rates.

Another group participating in this developing national pastime in the US are those who identify different ethnic and other groups with low caesarean rates and recommend the application of their practices in the USA. An example has been mentioned already in the context of Irish maternity care (section 4.2.8) where the National Maternity Hospital's low caesarean rates have contributed to the development of the doula industry in the USA (Mander, 2001a). A not dissimilar example is found in the research and recommendations by a certified nurse-midwife and an epidemiologist (Mahoney and Halinka Malcoe, 2005). These researchers used a case-control design to assess care in a Native American maternity unit in New Mexico. A caesarean rate of 9.6 per cent was identified. The researchers suggest that demographic factors, such as high parity and young maternal age, were largely responsible for these outcomes. They further identify cultural factors as influential, such as the avoidance of epidural analgesia. A further factor which was significantly associated with the birth outcome was the discipline of the attendant at the birth. Of the 137 obstetrician attended low-risk labours, 13 women (9.5 per cent) underwent a caesarean. Among the nurse-midwife attended group the figure was 39 out of 635 women (6.1 per cent). For this reason, these researchers recommend that 'non-obstetrician' (2005:177) care providers may lower caesarean rates in other populations too. The obvious flaws in the logic of this argument, though, may detract from the significance of the message.

4.3 Discussion – a UK perspective of the international issues

This overview of the international caesarean situation has underscored a number of important issues, some of which recur in several of the countries mentioned. That the United Kingdom has not been included in the sample of countries is a deliberate decision. This omission will be addressed in this general discussion of the issues raised, by adopting a UK orientation and drawing on relevant UK literature. For some of the issues, though, a UK-wide view may not be available. In this case, literature from one or more of the four countries which make up the UK will be used. This is likely to draw attention to some interesting and potentially important differences.

4.3.1 Demographics

With a population of about 60 million, the UK's GDP is positioned below that of France, but higher than Belgium's. That the UK National Health Service (NHS) provides 'health on the cheap' is evidenced by the relatively small proportion of the GDP being spent on health, compared with countries like France, Germany and, most notably, the USA. This limited spending may be contrasted with the fairly comprehensive service provision (OECD, 2003). In terms of the caesarean rate, in England it has continued to rise inexorably to reach 22.7 per cent in 2004; this figure is made up of 9.6 per cent elective and 13.1 per cent emergency caesareans. In Scotland, the health system has traditionally been criticised for being 'over doctored'; that this is so is supported by its caesarean rate always having been higher than England's, and having reached 24.4 per cent (ISD, 2004). While the Scottish elective caesarean rate rose to 9.0 per cent in 2003–04, the emergency rate remained static at the disconcertingly high level of 15.4 per cent. In both Scotland and England, the declining spontaneous birth rates balance the rising overall caesarean rates, whereas the falling forceps rate is balanced by the reciprocally rising rate of vacuum assisted births. To facilitate international comparisons, in 2004 the Scottish infant mortality rate was 49.6 per 10,000 population (ISD, 2005a).

4.3.2 Issues on the fringe

The benefits of being a country with a small geographical area emerged as significant in maintaining a high standard of maternity services in the Netherlands. On the other hand, the geographical problems of access to maternity services appeared to be just one of the challenges facing childbearing women in low-income countries. In the UK, as well as the major conurbations, there are large tracts of sparsely populated countryside, whose situation may best be described as 'rural and remote'. A number of initiatives, such as RURARI (the Remote and Rural Areas Resource Initiative), have been introduced to combat the typically poorer health among rural populations (Godden, 2005). Similarly, attempts have been made to address the challenges faced by rural childbearing women and their families (Tucker et al, 2005; McGuire et al, 2004).

A number of technological innovations, such as video conferencing, have been introduced to overcome the challenges of providing antenatal care to isolated families (SCC, 2001); the provision of appropriate care around and during the labour and birth, however, remains problematical. Perhaps as a result of these problems, for at least two decades the caesarean rates for the Scottish islands (Orkney, Shetland, Western Isles) have been disconcertingly higher than those of the mainland of Scotland (SPCERH, 2005).

4.3.3 Days and times

The finding in Israel (section 4.2.5) of not only elective but also emergency caesareans being undertaken at the 'convenience' of the operator appears scarcely believable (Cohain and Yoselis, 2004). To find that a parallel phenomenon exists in the UK is disconcerting. A national audit shows a fairly predictable decrease in the number of elective caesareans at weekends in Scotland (McIlwaine et al, 1998). Perhaps also for reasons of postnatal ward staffing, the number of elective caesareans is reduced on Fridays by almost one third. The pattern of emergency caesareans, though, follows a not dissimilar though less extreme pattern. The number of emergency operations falls by approximately 20 per cent at weekends. It is possible that these similarities are associated with a decrease in the number of women having labour induced at weekends although, with the declining induction rate, this association should be becoming less marked.

As well as the Scottish daily rate of caesareans mirroring the Israeli rate, it beggars belief that the Scottish pattern of the timing of caesarean should too. McIlwaine and her colleagues found, as would be expected, that a clear majority (54.6 per cent, n=1,779) of elective operations were performed between 09.00 and 12.00. The time when the lowest number of elective caesareans were undertaken was 03.00–06.00 (0.6 per cent, n=18). These researchers explain that these are likely to have been what I have termed 'emergency elective' operations (see section 3.1.1). The finding of a 'diurnal' or 'circadian' pattern of emergency operations, like that observed in Israel (Goldstick et al, 2003), was less predictable. McIlwaine and her colleagues found that the pattern of emergency caesareans followed that of elective operations, but with a slight time lag. Whereas elective operations peaked at 09.00–12.00, emergencies peaked at 12.00–15.00 (13.4 per cent, n=683). The time when fewest emergency caesareans were performed was 06.00–09.00 (8.1 per cent, n=415). These leave the observer with the disturbing impression that many of these emergency operations are something less than that and, as observed in Israel, operator convenience is a significant factor in the timing of emergency caesarean births.

4.3.4 Attitudes to caesarean

When considering the international picture, the impact of cultural developments on attitudes towards caesarean became apparent in a number of developed and less developed countries. It is possible that certain cultural changes may be occurring in the UK, although the research literature on this topic has yet to be generated. The cultural phenomena which may be happening relate to the well-recognised tendency of some women or couples to postpone childbearing. As has been shown by research, many women who embark on motherhood in their late thirties often do so because they have careers which are important to them (Berryman and Windridge, 1995). It may be suggested that such responsible careers carry a considerable degree of control over their own and others' lives. 'Letting go' of such control may prove difficult. A certain loss of control is inevitable in the context of motherhood, and early examples are those particularly uncontrollable phenomena, the onset and duration of labour. I venture to suggest that a woman who is accustomed to being in control of herself and others may seek to assume control over the birth of her baby. It may be that caesarean is one way for her to achieve such a degree of control. For this reason a woman may, for cultural reasons, endeavour to apply the attitudes and expectations which are inherent in her work life to her experience of motherhood.

4.3.5 *Private health care and socio-economic status*

The international comparisons demonstrate the powerful positive correlation in a number of countries between the caesarean rate and the prevalence of private health care. The reasons for this correlation have been shown to relate to culture, the quality of the public health system, insurance-led health care and/or entrepreneurial medical practitioners. In the UK, private health care forms a relatively small component, comprising only 16.6 per cent of health care expenditure (WHO, 2005). This may be the reason why it attracts so little attention in relation to UK caesarean rates. It is necessary to question, though, whether any other countries' issues relating to private health care apply in the UK. To examine this question I would suggest that, in many ways, socio-economic status (SES) may serve as a proxy for that section of the population who, in other countries, might be in a position to purchase private health care. For this reason, I consider here the relationship between UK caesarean rates and SES.

A potentially important exception to my observation of little attention given to private maternity care is found in County Armagh in Northern Ireland (SHSSC, 2000). In an environment featuring a somewhat medicalised system of maternity care (McCrea, 1996), it is not uncommon for women to pay an obstetrician to provide private antenatal care. This arrangement applies only to the pregnancy, so the intention is for these women to receive standard (NHS) care in labour. The reality, however, is quite different. Among women who had private antenatal care, the elective caesarean rate is almost three times the rate of women who had NHS care during pregnancy. Further, the emergency caesarean rate is 25 per cent higher, which the authors attribute to the higher rate of induction among women who had private antenatal care (SHSSC, 2000:51). Interventions in labour are not the only ones to be used more frequently. Rates of ultrasound scans are also higher (Robinson, 2000). The reasons for this increase in interventions are not clear. It is possible to surmise that against a backdrop of a culture of medicalisation, these pregnant women do not meet midwives, who would inform them of the evidence relating to the benefits of uncomplicated birth. Thus, the women's lack of confidence in their own ability to give birth spontaneously is likely to be reinforced by solely medical contact during pregnancy.

In England, caesarean rates were able to be analysed according to women's affluence. This involved Hospital Episode Statistics for caesarean being subjected to analysis using a multiple deprivation index based on electoral ward of residence (Barley et al, 2004). These researchers found that women in the least deprived categories, that is, the women residing in the more affluent areas, were significantly more likely to undergo an elective caesarean than women living in the other, more deprived, area. These findings have been challenged on methodological grounds (Macfarlane, 2004), but Barley and her colleagues do acknowledge that electoral wards are not homogeneous, and so some women would be wrongly categorised. Nevertheless, these researchers consider that their findings support the observations already mentioned regarding other countries. Thus, far from being 'too posh to push', the most deprived group may be 'too proletarian for caesarean' (2004:1399). Barley and colleagues' findings are endorsed by an analysis of public health statistics in the north west of England (NWPH, 2005). NWPH, though, analysed individuals' data, rather than electoral wards. Like Barley and her colleagues, NWPH reached the conclusion that caesarean rates show a strong 'inverse relationship with deprivation' (NWPH, 2005:17). This suggests that the overwhelming impression created in a large number of other countries also applies to the UK.

While some UK observers find the escalating caesarean rates disconcerting and the link with private medicine obnoxious, others perceive the situation differently. The longstanding fiscal problems of the NHS have, in a Machiavellian way, been linked to the general and evidence-based movement towards 'normal' childbearing. The result of this weirdly distorted thinking is the suggestion that the focus on normality is nothing more than a fiendishly clever money-saving scam (Revill, 2006). Such journalistic imaginings barely deserve mention, let alone further comment.

4.3.6 'Normal' childbearing

In my examination of the international caesarean situation (please see section 4.2 above), the input of the midwife in some countries was most noticeable by its near-absence. In China, the decline and fall of the midwife was documented, while her title was assumed by labour ward nurses (Cheung et al, 2005a). In Brazil, the midwife was found to be too low status to be employable (Nuttall, 2000). In Greece, only nurses were mentioned in the available research and other literature (Mossialos et al, 2005). All of these countries have seriously spiralling caesarean rates and the midwife only features for the purpose of being excluded from the equation. In the literature on the low-income countries, where the caesarean situation is complicated, the midwife never appears in the research or statistical literature.

Does it matter that there is no reference to the midwife in these countries where caesarean rates are widely recognised as becoming a major public health problem? I would argue that it does. This is because the country in which the midwife is most powerful is able to boast one of the lowest caesarean rates. This country is the Netherlands (Declercq and Viisainen, 2001). This view is supported by findings in the USA, a country with severe anxieties about its caesarean rates, where data clearly show that 'non-obstetrician care' (Mahoney and Malcoe, 2005:177) is fundamentally important to address the caesarean problem.

The way in which the midwife may influence the international caesarean problem may follow the example of the Dutch midwife. The culture in the Netherlands focuses on ensuring that childbearing remains as near 'normal' as possible. This aim, mentioned already in section 1.4.8, has been imported into the UK, where the midwife has long regarded herself as the 'guardian of normality' (Downe, 2004:173). Downe does not consider that this claim is entirely justified, because of the midwife's collusion with medical practitioners to convert childbearing into a technological experience, rather than a bio-psycho-social one. While Downe's criticisms are well founded, and it may be that many UK midwives have transformed themselves into *medwives*, there remains the infrastructure in place for midwives to practise *genuine* midwifery. As Wagner observes, whether and to what extent midwives lower the caesarean rate is related to their autonomy in their practice (2002). Reassurance may be drawn from the fact that some midwives are already practising genuinely autonomously, particularly those in independent practice.

The effect of genuine midwifery practice on the caesarean rate is demonstrated by the statistics collected by the Independent Midwives Association (IMA). For this albeit small group of practitioners the caesarean rate is 13.6 per cent (n=46/337) (IMA, 2005). For a large proportion of the independent midwife's clients, like those of the Dutch midwife, the home is where she chooses to give birth. As has been shown in section 3.3.1.1, the link between place of birth and caesarean may be something more than just a matter of coincidence.

4.4 Conclusion

In this chapter, I have examined the international picture of caesarean. The problems associated with defining an appropriate caesarean rate are clearly apparent. The escalating rates and the likely causative factors have been identified. The inappropriate use of caesarean is associated with health systems which operate on an entrepreneurial basis. Unnecessary caesareans are iatrogenic, to the extent of increasing maternal morbidity and mortality rates. Inappropriate caesarean provision, which may actually include the non-availability of the operation, is a particular problem in countries where maternal death is a major public health issue. I have suggested that generally rising caesarean rates reflect a trend away from expectations of normal or uncomplicated childbearing. Strategies to remedy this trend have arisen out of the research literature and statistics.

5 Caesarean decision making – who's choosing the choices?

The ownership of the decision for a woman to undergo or not undergo a caesarean is fiercely disputed. The main protagonists in the dispute are probably the woman and the person who may perform the operation. In spite of this, any number of other parties have (at least) a passing interest in this decision. As well as who makes the decision, the method of deciding and the basis on which the decision is reached are also highly contentious. Caesarean decision making inevitably revolves around individual or clinical interactions. There are, however, other levels of decisions which will undoubtedly impact on those made at the interpersonal level. These other levels also warrant attention. Thus, in many settings and at many levels, decision making in the context of caesarean deserves close and careful consideration.

5.1 Dynamics of decision making

I have already outlined some major categories of indications or reasons for the caesarean operation (see section 3.2). They were classified broadly according to problems for the mother, problems for the baby and problems for both. In that section, while demonstrating some of the possibilities, I attempted to suggest that the indications for a surgical birth are in no way absolute, fixed or immutable. The criteria for the caesarean operation vary over time and according to a range of factors, including the existence of research evidence, the availability of necessary technology and the accessibility of appropriate clinical skills. As well as caesarean decisions varying over a long time scale, there is also the potential for them to change more speedily. Rapid changes might occur due to alterations in the environment, such as staffing, or in the condition of the woman or the baby.

There is also the potential for caesarean decisions, which are inevitably subjective, to vary within an individual as well as between individuals. Examples would include the effects of expert knowledge and occupational and personal experience. I would also suggest that, as in some other childbearing and caring decisions, gut feeling and intuition may have a part to play. It is possible that decisions are affected by general attitudes too, such as those promulgated by the media, be they public or professional (please see section 1.4.7). This raises the likelihood that fashion may be a contributing factor. Of course, the decision is likely to be at least influenced by who makes it, as this will unavoidably reflect their orientation and personal or occupational background.

A problem which invariably impedes any decision making is the lack of knowledge of future consequences. In caesarean decision making this problem applies particularly to possible risks; although some involved in the decision will be aware of such risks, the extent to which they divulge them to the other parties is uncertain. These future consequences may introduce the need for a, possibly unforeseen, cascade of subsequent decisions. Thus, the complexity of this developing process is compounded, and has been summarised as:

> ill-structured problems, uncertain dynamic environments, shifting, ill-defined, or competing goals, action/feedback loops, time stress, high stakes, multiple players, organisational goals and norms.
>
> (Orasanu and Connolly, 1993:7)

For these reasons, the complex nature of caesarean decision making and its context demand that it should be approached as the dynamic phenomenon which it undoubtedly is (Hedberg and Larsson, 2004).

5.2 Clinical, interpersonal and individual decision making

Because of its ubiquity and immediacy, I consider first the context of the decision making which happens on an interpersonal basis between individuals. These decisions may often be taken in a clinical setting, such as at an antenatal check, in a birthing room in the labour ward or in the operating department. They are preceded, however, by deliberations and possibly decisions located in less formal settings. Although these discussions may happen in, for example, the woman's home, they are no less important.

5.2.1 Context

The context serves as the broad framework or backdrop to decision making. The importance of its influence on the process and the outcome is not to be underestimated.

5.2.1.1 Autonomy

The fundamental significance of personal and occupational autonomy in decision making, such as that preceding caesarean, should not need to be stated. The reality, however, may be somewhat different from the rhetoric. There is a distinct possibility that the woman's autonomy will be limited, first, by the choices which are actually presented to her (Mander, 1993b) and, second, by her access to relevant information (McLeod and Sherwin, 2000). Both of these prerequisites are likely to be under the control, initially, of the midwife, who may consider some decisions inappropriate for the woman and some information outwith the woman's comprehension.

Alternatively, or perhaps additionally, the midwife's autonomy in information giving may be proscribed if she works in a 'rule-bound, risk culture' which may be a feature of some health care organisations (Edwards, 2003). Because of the nature of the environment of midwifery care, both the woman and the midwife may find themselves having to employ devious strategies which will help them to avoid confrontation with 'the system', while still maintaining some degree of personal and occupational integrity.

5.2.1.2 Culture

The devious strategies, just mentioned, reflect the relationship between the midwife and the NHS institution by which she is likely to be employed. This relationship clearly demonstrates the tension for the midwife whose prime concern is to be 'with woman' (Kirkham, 1999). In order to achieve this crucial midwifery function, there has evolved a form of practice known as 'doing good by stealth' (Kirkham, 1999:736) to which the conscientious midwife may have to resort. The institutions into which birth has been removed, that is hospitals, are characterised by the ethos of the dominant occupational group to ensure centralisation and efficiency. These stereotypically masculine attributes contrast with the characteristics crucial to midwives, including communicating, providing support and 'being with'. Thus, the cultural milieu in which the woman is expected to make decisions relating to her childbearing is peopled with disciplines whose occupational assumptions are diametrically opposed. These contrasting positions are further compounded by the perception of some obstetricians, among others, of a clear hierarchical relationship. In considering such relationships, Wagner (2000) recounts the marginalisation of the midwife and her practice in settings where medical power is greatest. These are the countries where medical hegemony is endorsed by private practice and other cultural factors, to produce the escalating caesarean rates discussed in Chapter 4. Wagner is scathingly critical of inappropriate medical involvement. By way of illustration, he draws a comparison between the practices of having an obstetric surgeon attend normal births with permitting only paediatric surgeons to act as babysitters to healthy toddlers.

5.2.1.3 Assumptions

The inter-occupational distinctions in maternity are aggravated by differing frames of reference, but likewise, assumptions may be made about what the woman prefers. LoCicero (1993) observes how stereotypes may be used to bypass the inconvenience of potentially uncomfortable and time-consuming questions and answers. She contemplates the likelihood of misunderstandings, when engaging in open discussion is not a priority for the obstetrician providing prenatal care. Such poor communication means that the woman's 'expectations, hopes and beliefs . . . are significantly compromised by the labor and birth process' (1993:1262).

When the woman is disappointed by her experience of the processes of labour and birth, she tends to blame herself, her body or her baby, for letting her down.

This self-blame persists for a variable period of time. It certainly lasts longer than her postnatal stay in the maternity unit, during which time she may try to convince herself and others that the outcome was 'for the best' under the circumstances. Her self-blame is likely to extend beyond her discharge from the maternity services. The woman's delayed realisation of where responsibility for her experience lies means that when it dawns she may no longer be in contact with those responsible. Thus, there is no opportunity to give them feedback. This means that the personnel involved continue in blissful ignorance of the woman's perceptions of their behaviour. This ignorance may actually serve to fuel the beliefs of those who provide care, particularly regarding the accuracy and relevance of the medical model which they espouse.

5.2.1.4 Gender issues

The significance of gender in maternity decision making is arguably becoming more complex. LoCicero even suggests that the increasing numbers of females being accepted into medical schools means that eventually the numbers of females and males in medicine, and hence the gender balance, will be equal (1993). The fallacy of this argument may be found in the gendered nature of medicine. This is an occupational group in which the women entrants who seek advancement are required to curb their stereotypically female characteristics and assume more 'masculine' ones (Stephens, 1998; Mander, 2004a). Thus, LoCicero's optimism is clearly misplaced, although even she questions whether women will ever be in a position to challenge the status quo. She goes on to recognise the indubitably gendered nature of the medical model of care (see section 5.2.2.2.2 below). LoCicero argues that the attributes which I have referred to as 'stereotypical' are considerably more than that. She draws on cross-cultural psychological findings to explain the willingness of women to 'conform, defer and comply' with expert advice, whereas men 'are more likely to express dominance over females' (1993:1266). Although such views may be far from politically correct, the behaviour which they represent may actually be quite familiar.

5.2.1.5 Power

The hegemony of the medical model in childbearing means that the midwife is forced in her practice and decision making to allow herself either to become marginalised (Wagner, 2000) or else to become an adherent of it. If she chooses the latter route she puts herself in danger of becoming that chameleon of caring – the '*medwife*'. While appearing to be a bona fide midwife, the medwife practices and makes decisions in accordance with the patriarchal medical power structure. The ability of the medwife to provide support for a woman, who is at risk of subordination by the personnel and institution where she is giving birth, is limited to the point of being non-existent. Thus, both the childbearing woman and the medwife are effectively disempowered by the institution. The body of the childbearing woman serves as one arena in which this power play is acted out (Edwards,

2005). If, as Edwards argues, the positioning of a stethoscope is a manifestation of the power relationship, how much more evident is this power in the birth of the baby by the caesarean operation?

5.2.1.6 Choice

By way of denying the existence of this imbalance of power in childbearing decision making, critics argue the voluntary nature and women's willing acceptance of, for example, the medicalised approach to birth. Such choice is little more than illusory, with lip service featuring prominently (Beech, 2003). In reality that choice is, at best, unrecognised and more likely rhetorical to the point of non-existence. UK maternity policy-makers have articulated the rhetoric of choice since the Winterton Report (HoC, 1992) advocated the 'three Cs' (choice, control and continuity). But realisation has gradually dawned that empty rhetoric is the sum total of what child-bearing women are being offered.

In her perceptive analysis of the availability of childbearing choices within the UK maternity services, Edwards (2003) highlights the ubiquity of the dominance of the medical model of care. As mentioned already (section 5.2.1.1), practitioners limit the woman's autonomy by controlling the choices available to her. While this is done, presumably, with the best of intentions, there is no way that a woman is able to make her own decisions under such circumstances. Thus, as Richards apocryphally portrayed childbearing choice in 1982, there is no point in offering the woman frozen cod or frozen haddock when what she is seeking is fresh fish. On this basis, Edwards argues that childbearing decision making should recognise and possibly even celebrate differences. This will ensure that the 'diverse beliefs about birth' (2003:11) will be catered for via a multiplicity of dialogues, through which choice will eventually begin to emerge from the realms of rhetoric.

The role of the childbearing woman and her midwife attendant in making the caesarean decision, thus, appears to be somewhat circumscribed.

5.2.2 Indications and thresholds

I have argued already that caesarean decision making is a dynamic process. In this section, I examine that dynamism in terms of its variability over an extended time period. In this instance, the time period may run into decades. The link between dynamism and decision making is due to the indications or reasons for performing a caesarean, which have been discussed previously (please see section 3.2). The burden of the argument in this section is that the caesarean rate fluctuates, or more accurately rises, in association with a range of factors which have the effect of moving the threshold of what the decision-makers consider appropriate (Weaver, 2004:1). Hence, the decision about whether to perform the operation also differs. The result is that processes, which at one point in time are deemed to be satisfactory, physiological and safe, may be moved to the other side of the 'threshold of appropriateness'. For this reason the same processes are viewed quite differently and suddenly cease to be physiological. In the present context, the other side of that threshold means that the phenomenon is transformed into being an indication for caesarean. The movement of perceptions of these processes in this way is brought about by a range of factors, some of which are explicit and tangible; others are less so. Thus, I propose that the dynamic nature of decision making involves what is effectively a movement of the goal posts, or of the assumptions on which the caesarean decision is founded.

This dynamic mobility of the thresholds of caesarean decisions involves not only the medical decision-makers. It involves all of the interested parties, but because the caesarean decision is primarily medical, that needs to be the main focus of this debate.

These dynamic processes have been facilitated to some extent by the classification of caesarean decision making recognised by Francome and his colleagues (1993). These authors show that the indications for the operation may be 'relative' (1993:65) or 'absolute' (1993:60). They maintain that the absolute indications are those situations in which caesarean is the 'only safe option' for the woman, the baby or both. They argue that cephalo-pelvic disproportion, intrauterine growth retardation (IUGR), placenta praevia and eclampsia are absolute indications. I venture to suggest, however, that, with the exception of eclampsia, these conditions constitute relative indications, particularly if their variable severity is considered. Additionally, the recognition of these conditions may vary according to the technology being used and there may also be a possibility of the duration of pregnancy or the onset of labour affecting their continuing presence. These supposedly 'absolute' indications are discussed in more detail below.

Francome and his colleagues also draw attention to the 'relative' indications for caesarean. By this, they mean certain conditions which are less precisely defined, such as 'fetal distress' and 'failure to progress', or 'dystocia' as it may be known in the USA. Quite appropriately, these authors relate the escalation in the number of caesareans performed for these conditions to the medicalisation of childbearing. I consider below, though, whether there may be other factors which are also involved. These factors may include a greater unwillingness or unpreparedness, for a variety of reasons, to accept even a small risk of harm to the mother, or more particularly, to the baby. It may be that this unwillingness may expose the mother to the greater risk of caesarean for the sake of a considerably lesser risk to the baby. But, because that lesser risk is perceived as unacceptable, the greater risk is not discussed and may even be disregarded. A similar argument is traced in an account of how, as the caesarean operation became safer in the late twentieth century and the spectre of maternal death receded, the operation's apparent advantages to the fetus 'became ever more seductive' (Penn and Ghaem-Maghami, 2001:1). As I have observed already, when the operation is undertaken for fetal reasons, the benefits which are conferred on the baby are, if quantified at all, negligible (Penn and Ghaem-Maghami, 2001). Conversely, these authors point out that the considerably greater risks of the caesarean operation to the woman are far less likely to be taken into account. This, they argue, is in spite of caesarean's 'four to five fold' (2001:2) increase in maternal mortality compared with a vaginal birth. This argument is taken to its logical conclusion when the authors draw attention to the acknowledged way that women, in the interests of the baby, may expose themselves to additional and possibly unnecessary risks to their own life and health. On this basis Penn and Ghaem-Maghami go on to argue the need for better information on which women may base such momentous decisions.

5.2.2.1 The 'absolute' indications

The indications for caesarean which Francome and his colleagues classify as 'absolute' (1993:60) comprise cephalo-pelvic disproportion, intrauterine growth retardation (IUGR), placenta praevia and eclampsia. With the last condition there is probably little alternative to caesarean if the woman and baby are to survive. If we assume that eclampsia is correctly diagnosed, it is a condition which is either present or absent. The woman either has an eclamptic fit or she doesn't, there are no gradations. Thus, the assertion made by Francome and colleagues is appropriate. The other three conditions, though, vary hugely in their severity from the mildly inconvenient to the life threatening. Like many others, the diagnosis of these conditions is neither easy nor consistent. These problems relate not only to the diagnosis, but also to the interventions to remedy such conditions.

5.2.2.1.1 CEPHALO-PELVIC DISPROPORTION

This means simply that this particular baby's head is too large to pass through this particular woman's pelvis at this particular time. While this may give the impression of being easily diagnosed, estimation of the size of the baby and of the pelvis is not yet a precise science. Nor is it possible to calculate in advance the extent to which the fetal head will 'mould', in order to negotiate the mother's pelvis, or the extent to which the mother's pelvic joints will 'give' during labour. So, although a diagnosis of either 'fetal macrosomia' (big baby) or 'contracted pelvis' may sound persuasive, the reality is based on not very much. As Garrey and colleagues observed some time ago, it is not possible to diagnose cephalo-pelvic disproportion until 'labour has been in progress for some time' (1969:257). Thus, making an accurate diagnosis of cephalo-pelvic disproportion prior to established labour is not feasible. This is partly because after labour begins a number of other factors are brought into play.

5.2.2.1.2 INTRAUTERINE GROWTH RETARDATION (IUGR)

IUGR, or fetal growth restriction, is routinely screened for during antenatal checks by measuring the distance in centimetres between the woman's symphysis pubis and the fundus of her uterus. The accuracy of such subjective measurements is a source of concern. The only research into this investigation (Lindhard et al, 1990) is limited in its scope and the topic needs to be revisited. Thus, the initial screening for IUGR is less than reliable. Further, the reliability of ultrasound, which is used to confirm the diagnosis, is dependent on the skill of the ultrasonographer.

5.2.2.1.3 PLACENTA PRAEVIA

Placenta praevia, when the placenta is partially or wholly situated in the lower segment of the uterus, may be a cause of haemorrhage sufficient to threaten the woman's life. In the most severe type, the risk of haemorrhage is compounded by the placenta effectively occluding the cervix and preventing the baby from being born. As well as this most severe degree of placenta praevia, there are lesser degrees, which may be so mild that the placenta barely impinges on the lower segment. Additionally, although a severe degree may be diagnosed by ultrasound early in pregnancy, the differential growth and expansion rates of the different parts of the uterus mean that this problem may have disappeared by the onset of labour at term (Chama et al, 2004).

5.2.2.1.4 OTHER 'ABSOLUTE' INDICATIONS

Other 'absolute' indications have been said to include transverse lie in labour or severe placental abruption. It may be, though, that the risks of these conditions are also relative. In the case of transverse lie, for example, the variation is associated with both the size, or gestational age, of the baby and the size of the woman's pelvis.

5.2.2.2 The 'relative' indications

The current seriously risk-averse nature of the maternity services is partly responsible for the changing thresholds and the increasing number of caesareans being performed for the relative indications; by which is meant those that are 'more loosely defined' (Francome et al, 1993). The examples to which Francome and his colleagues refer comprise fetal distress and failure to progress in labour. I suggest, though, that there are a number of other conditions which, although not 'loosely defined', are the subject of considerable debate about whether and to what extent they are actually indications for caesarean.

5.2.2.2.1 FETAL DISTRESS

Fetal distress is a presumption of fetal compromise due to fetal hypoxia or a reduction in the oxygen supply to the fetus. It is the major indication in approximately one quarter of caesareans (Thomas and Paranjothy, 2001:48). In such situations, the caesarean would be undertaken to 'rescue' the fetus from what is thought to be a hostile intrauterine environment. The assumption is that, if the baby were to remain *in utero*, the lack of oxygen might cause the death of at least some fetal cells, such as those of the brain. The diagnosis of fetal distress is commonly made by the routine use of continuous electronic fetal monitoring (CEFM) when the woman is in labour. This form of monitoring has been condemned for being a major cause of the escalating caesarean rates. Thus, the benefits, or otherwise, of routine CEFM have been the subject of many research projects and fierce debates.

In their authoritative systematic review of the randomised controlled trials (see section 3.2.1.2), Thacker and his colleagues (2001) found thirteen published trials which focused on the safety and the efficiency of CEFM. The trials compared the condition of babies who had been monitored in labour using CEFM with those monitored using intermittent auscultation, by either a Pinards or Doppler. Of the thirteen trials, only nine were of a good enough standard to be included in Thacker and colleagues' systematic review. The only benefit to be identified, which was statistically significant, was the reduced likelihood of babies who had been monitored by CEFM succumbing to a seizure or fit in the neonatal period. There were no significant differences in the babies' condition at birth or their admission for neonatal intensive care. Although a fit or seizure may sound alarming for a newborn baby, it is not the dreadful problem that it may appear. The limited severity of the problem is demonstrated by the fact that even though more of the non-CEFM babies had fits, neither the perinatal mortality rate nor the cerebral palsy rate was increased among these babies. On the other hand, Thacker and his colleagues found that, as mentioned already, both the caesarean rate and the assisted vaginal delivery rate were significantly increased when CEFM was used.

In view of the serious implications of interpretation, it may be surprising that there is a not inconsiderable element of subjectivity in interpreting the CEFM printout or 'strip'. This subjectivity was identified as long ago as 1978 (Trimbos and Keirse). These researchers found not only inter-rater variability (between observers), but also intra-rater variability (in the same observer) over time. That these failings persist has been shown by work on midwives' interpretation (Devane and Lalor, 2005). It may be suggested, though, that midwives may not be unique in the continuing subjectivity of their interpretation.

In a systematic review of electrocardiography in labour, observation is made of the association between routine CEFM and unnecessary interventions, such as emergency caesarean (Neilson, 2003). He does suggest, though, that the use of fetal blood sampling (FBS) to confirm the presence of fetal distress, when there is a non-reassuring CEFM printout, may reduce the number of unnecessary interventions. Although fetal blood sampling is a decidedly unpleasant investigation for the woman, it may be one way of avoiding a needless caesarean without putting at risk the well-being of the baby. The extent to which FBS is actually employed is demonstrated in a survey auditing caesarean (Thomas and Paranjothy, 2001). These researchers found that in only a minority (49.6 per cent) of maternity units was FBS even possible. Of these maternity units, in an even smaller minority (43.6 per cent) was this investigation actually used to assess the condition of the baby before undertaking the caesarean.

Neilson goes on to advocate the use of an electrocardiograph (ECG) trace in the event of a non-reassuring CEFM result. My occupational experience leads me to suggest that the 'clip' on the baby's scalp may not be a reliable form of monitoring. Additionally, it also carries the risk of the exchange of body fluids between the mother and her baby.

Thus, it is apparent that there are a number of issues to take into account when considering the diagnosis of fetal distress as an indication for caesarean. This brief examination shows that this indication is certainly relative, as Francome and his colleagues suggested in 1993.

5.2.2.2.2 FAILURE TO PROGRESS

Failure to progress is a seriously unfortunate diagnostic label to be applied to a woman in labour. Its negative connotations are equalled by terms such as 'incompetent cervix' and 'habitual abortion'. This term's North American equivalent, 'dystocia', is no more acceptable or precise, being translated as just 'difficult labour'. The term 'dystocia' was used by Victorian obstetricians in Scotland to indicate insufficient or inadequate uterine contractions. These meanings and origins lead to the inevitable question 'Difficult for whom?' Then as now, the woman's contractions could 'go off' for a range of reasons. Similarly, then as now, some of these reasons were related to pharmacological and other interventions, that is, they were iatrogenic (Mander, 1998). The extent of the problem of failure to progress has been shown in the finding that one fifth of caesareans are performed for this indication. The majority (60 per cent) of women being diagnosed are first time mothers (Thomas and Paranjothy, 2001).

Whether and to what extent this concept is appropriate as an indication for caesarean does need careful attention. Francome and colleagues' label of failure to progress as a relative indication for caesarean is probably correct. This is because this concept has followed on from the related and more absolute term 'prolonged labour'. Such a labour could be defined in a number of ways, usually related to duration; perhaps most notoriously in the injunction not to 'let the sun set twice on the same labour' (Llewellyn-Jones, 1969:300). Making a diagnosis of prolonged labour was challenging and arbitrary, relying as it did on the all too often unknown timing of the onset or establishment of labour.

Both the difficulty of making the diagnosis and the frequency of it were intended to be reduced by the introduction of the partograph (see section 4.1.1). This diagrammatic form of documentation of the woman's progress in labour originally sought to facilitate intervention in advance of any serious deterioration in the woman's condition or in that of her baby. The partograph which, like so many inventions, began as comparatively benign, soon developed its own momentum. Thus, this diagrammatic representation of the woman's progress, and more specifically that of her cervix, has taken on a life of its own. It has ceased to be just a record which serves to benefit women and babies by reducing maternal and perinatal mortality and morbidity. Through the partograph, the technological imperative has manifested itself, by which a beneficial intervention evolves into a doctrine or dogma, requiring observance and adherence. In this way, the partograph appears to have effectively developed teeth with which it requires that women and their attendants are obliged to follow slavishly the alert line and the action line. Thus, the dogma of the partograph is 'rarely questioned' (Groeschel and Glover, 2001:22).

In the same way that questioning the dogma of the partograph is not permitted, deviation from its ethos may also not be permitted. The fundamental principle which is encapsulated in the partograph is the incrementalist concept of continuous progress in the woman's labour. Such progress may be measured during vaginal examination in the changes in the cervix and descent of the presenting part. The findings are recorded on the graph in the partograph. These incrementalist assumptions of the progress of labour derive from research by Friedman in 1954.

He attempted to provide a graphic representation of progress in labour and produced a diagram which has become known as 'Friedman's Curve'. This diagram,
though, is based on Friedman's monitoring of the progress of a small (n=100) but
heterogeneous group of labouring women by means of rectal examinations. The
precise time of onset of their labours was uncertain. Some of the women were
experiencing physiological labour, but others were experiencing complicated labour
due to fetal malpositions or malpresentations or they were having labour induced
or augmented or were receiving regional analgesia. All of these conditions are
likely to affect the progress of labour. This obviously seriously flawed research
resulted in the conclusion that the cervix dilates at the apocryphal rate of 'one
centimetre per hour for two hours'. Anyone who has ever experienced or attended
a woman in spontaneous uncomplicated labour knows that this myth bears
little relation to reality. If a woman is relaxed and in her own environment, labour
may discontinue and then resume according to what is happening in and around
the woman. Some of these pauses may be late and long, with no detriment to the
woman or the baby (Banks, 2000). Because of the flawed nature of his research,
and because some are able to see the reality of uncomplicated labour, Friedman's
work has been extensively criticised (Lavender, 2003; Zhang et al, 2002; Cesario,
2004).

It is clearly apparent that the standard which is used to measure the woman's
progress in labour is defective. The instrument, the partograph, against which her
performance is assessed, is based on imperfect data. LoCicero, however, argues
that this instrument reflects the masculine medical model, fitting, as it does, the
obstetrician's need 'to wrest control of the birth process' from the woman (1993:
1262). LoCicero goes on to discuss the possibility of psychological causes for the
woman's labour 'slowing down' (1993:1264). She, like Simkin and Ancheta (2000),
approach the labour from the viewpoint of the medical model needing to be confronted, but still assuming a fixed time for the various stages of labour. These views
are compounded by the assumption that the labour environment is somewhere other
than the woman's own home. These authors also draw on the literature on the effects
of anxiety on labour, quoting liberally the work of Odent (1993). His invention of
the 'fetus ejection reflex' adopts a similar stance, which seeks to pathologise any
variation in the progress of labour (Odent, 2004). The midwifery model, on the
other hand, would argue that the well-being of the mother and her baby are the
focus of interest, rather than what the clock dictates or any observations that are
recorded on a partograph.

While failure to progress may in itself be recorded as the main indication for a
caesarean, this diagnosis should be viewed as part of an ongoing process rather
than simply a chance event. An audit of caesarean in England, Wales and Northern
Ireland clearly shows the nature of this process (Thomas and Paranjothy, 2001).
In the various regions the number of women who had had oxytocin administered
to augment labour prior to a caesarean for failure to progress ranged from 84.6 per
cent in Northern Ireland to 74 per cent in the West Midlands. These figures clearly
demonstrate the part which failure to progress plays in the cascade of intervention
(see section 1.4.9). That failure to progress is part of an iatrogenic cascade shows

how little has changed since Victorian obstetricians recognised the concept and named it 'dystocia', perhaps because of the difficulty which it caused to them.

5.2.2.2.3 BREECH PRESENTATION AND BREECH BIRTH

The presentation of the baby with her foot, knee or buttocks lowest in the birth canal, or breech presentation, is likely to be regarded by some as an absolute indication for caesarean (Francome et al, 1993:70). This statement is one of the few certainties about breech presentation, and even it is subject to intense debate (see section 2.5.2). Often referred to as a 'malpresentation' because the baby has not adopted a cephalic presentation, the incidence of breech presentation varies according to a number of factors. In early pregnancy, almost 50 per cent of babies adopt a breech presentation but by term this proportion has reduced to about 3–4 per cent (RCOG, 2006:1). It may be argued that breech presentation and breech birth are abnormal and, thus, requiring medical attention. Such an argument has serious implications for women, their babies and their midwives (see section 5.2.2.2.3.2).

The 'abnormality' of a breech birth together with the well-rehearsed risks to the baby combine to create a persuasive argument that babies presenting by the breech should be born by caesarean. The success of this argument is apparent in the observation that breech presentation, along with dystocia, fetal compromise and repeat caesarean, has 'consistently' been one of the four major indications for caesarean (Thomas and Paranjothy, 2001). Although this argument is clearly successful, its basis in fact is quite a different matter. It may be that there are a number of factors operating, other than the welfare of the baby.

A North America-based research project, the Term Breech Trial (TBT) was intended to resolve these longstanding questions (Hannah et al, 2000). It was singularly unsuccessful in achieving these aims. Quite understandably, these authors presented their findings, which were overwhelmingly favourable to elective caesarean, as authoritative. Their publication, though, has raised more questions than it answered. These questions relate not only to the most appropriate way for a woman to give birth to her baby presenting as a breech, but also to the practice and interpretation of randomised controlled trials (Keirse, 2002; Kotaska, 2004) (please see section 2.5.2).

5.2.2.2.3.1 Attempts to 'remedy' a breech presentation   Paradoxically, in spite of their acceptance of the rather questionable findings of the Hannah and colleagues' study (2000), a Scottish expert advisory group still found it necessary to seek interventions by which to avoid caesareans for breech (SPCERH, 2001). Similarly, a number of systematic reviews have been undertaken to examine the methods by which caesarean may be avoided by converting the breech in to a cephalic presentation. This interest in the alternatives is surprising if the caesarean solution is as generally acceptable as its advocates would lead us to believe.

The research literature on using moxibustion, derived from Traditional Chinese Medicine (TCM), to cause the baby to move from being a breech presentation has been reviewed (Coyle et al, 2005). The reviewers conclude, though, that there is not yet sufficient evidence to make any firm recommendations. Similarly, encouraging the woman to adopt specific positions to cause the baby to move into a cephalic presentation has also been attempted (Hofmeyr and Kulier, 2000). Postures, such as the knee-chest position, though, have not yet been subjected to suitably large and rigorous study.

Offering External Cephalic Version (ECV) routinely at term to women with a breech presentation is by no means invariably successful. It has been shown to significantly reduce both the number of babies who are born other than head-first and the number of caesareans (Hofmeyr and Kulier, 2000). These reviewers found there to be no impact on perinatal mortality or morbidity. On the other hand, the use of ECV before term improves the outcome for neither the woman nor her baby (Hutton and Hofmeyr, 2006). While ECV at term is thought to carry fewer risks for the woman and the baby than caesarean, some women anecdotally report that ECV is a far from pleasant experience. The use of pain scales, though, suggests that women experience less pain if the ECV is successful (Fok et al, 2005). Further, it is a procedure that requires considerable manual dexterity on the part of the operator. There is thought to be the possibility of causing a minor degree of placental separation, which may engender Rhesus Haemolytic Disease in women who are Rhesus negative. Such placental separation, though, has been blamed on over-forceful manipulation (Hofmeyr and Gyte, 2004). It may be that such adverse outcomes, combined with the relatively increased safety of the caesarean operation, caused the practice of ECV to fall into disuse in the late twentieth century. Unsurprisingly, when such manual skills are not used or taught, they are soon likely to be lost.

Excessive tone or contractility of the uterine muscles is the main factor to have been blamed for ECV's limited success. For this reason, the use of medication to reduce the uterine tone has been recommended. Thus, drugs such as the betamimetics (salbutamol, ritodrine) may be administered prior to the ECV to achieve tocolysis; the ECV has been shown to be more likely to be successful if such medications are administered to prepare the woman (Hofmeyr and Gyte, 2004). On the basis of the research evidence, the Chief Medical Officer of Scotland was advised that a policy of offering routine ECV at term under tocolysis should be introduced (SPCERH, 2001). At the time of writing, the results of this initiative have not yet been made available.

5.2.2.2.3.2 The midwife's role As has been mentioned already (see section 1.4.8), the definition of what constitutes 'normal' childbearing has been increasingly manipulated to, effectively, reduce the likelihood of physiological birth. This has had the effect of, not only facilitating increased medical intervention in childbirth, but also limiting the role and scope of activity of the midwife. Her functions have been redefined by medical personnel to include only those activities which medical people perceive to be of little value, such as being with a woman during labour. While some midwives, some of whom have been referred to as 'medwives' (see section 4.3.6), have willingly accepted this limitation of their role, others have earnestly resisted such marginalisation.

Breech birth, like home birth, is one area in which such resistance is manifesting itself. There are a number of midwives who are confident to and skilled in attending a woman whose baby is presenting by the breech. Mary Cronk and Jane Evans are two such midwives, who have published their principles for caring for a woman experiencing a breech birth (Beech, 2003/04:6). These midwives emphasise the physiological nature of breech labour and birth. They also address the possibility that, in the event of labour becoming delayed, caesarean may still be advisable (Cronk, 2005:3). Cronk warns against the use of oxytocic drugs to drive this baby through the pelvis, or the use of 'actively managed breech extractions' (Beech, 2003/04:6) to drag the baby into this world. That midwives are the ideal people to assist breech births is attested by my own observation that the smoothest and most controlled breech birth that I have ever had the honour to witness was attended by a midwife.

It may be that midwives such as Mary Cronk and Jane Evans are effectively confronting the medical fraternity, through their preparedness to attend breech births. These midwives assist women in a birth which medical personnel, first, redefined as abnormal, thus placing it outwith the remit of the midwife. This birth was then further redefined as too hazardous, putting it beyond the scope of even medical practitioners. In this way vaginal breech birth has been made generally unavailable. Thus, this repeated redefinition impacted on both midwives and women and may be interpreted as an assumption of medical control extending far beyond the limits of medical decision making and practice. These strategies could easily be interpreted as a form of interprofessional domination. Such changes in obstetric practice are bound up with fear of litigation giving rise to defensive practice. Inadvertently, though, in the same way as medical skills in performing ECV disappeared in the late twentieth century, so too have the medical skills necessary to attend a breech birth. This disappearance is one of the few indisputable conclusions which emerged out of the Term Breech Trial (Hannah et al, 2000).

5.2.2.2.3.3 Maternal outcomes   In spite of the issues of medical deskilling, the major focus of the breech birth debate is indubitably the welfare of the baby; there is the potential for injuries or other harm to be sustained during the birth, or more likely the delivery (Beech, 2002a:4). While the well-being of the baby is clearly the woman's prime consideration, her own welfare also deserves consideration. As I have established elsewhere (please see Chapter 6), there are risks, albeit relatively infrequent, to the mother in giving birth by caesarean. Whether this information should be or is being imparted to women who are seeking to weigh up the relative benefits of caesarean versus vaginal breech birth is not clear.

5.2.2.2.3.3 Summary   The old advice to keep the 'Hands off the breech' has recently been resurrected (Cronk, 2005). It may be that the hands to be kept off are not only those near the breech as the presenting part as it distends the perineum and is born. But the hands to be kept off are also the medical hands which may be well advised, in order to give due acknowledgement to what is increasingly being recognised as an area of midwifery expertise.

5.2.2.2.4 MULTIPLE PREGNANCY

The link between multiple pregnancy and caesarean has become firmer as the 'twinning' rate has more than doubled in the past two decades (Botting, 1995; Barrett, 2004). Although the monozygotic (identical) twinning rate is stable at about 3.5 per 1,000 births, the greater use of assisted reproduction and the rising age of mothers has hugely increased dizygotic (fraternal) twinning and the higher multiple pregnancies (Dodd and Crowther, 2005). This latter observation means that, paradoxically, not only is there an escalation of the risks to all concerned, but also in the hopes and aspirations of couples who have previously been childless.

The risks of multiple pregnancy apply throughout the childbearing cycle. Because, however, the presentation of the second or subsequent babies is unpredictable after the vaginal birth of the first, the issues relating to multiple pregnancy may be not entirely dissimilar to those of the breech presentation (see section 5.2.2.2.3). The hazards of an unpredictable presentation, though, are compounded by the risks which may arise if there is a shared amniotic sac or any degree of twin-to-twin transfusion syndrome (Penn and Ghaem-Maghami, 2001).

A large retrospective epidemiological study of twin births was undertaken in Scotland, which showed that among the babies born at term, the outcomes for the second twin are significantly worse than those for the older sibling (Smith et al, 2002). In the case of the majority of the second twins who did not survive, the cause was found to be anoxia linked to mechanical problems, that is, delay due to malpresentation. The risk of asphyxia in the second baby increases markedly if the twin-twin delivery interval is more than 30 minutes (Dodd and Crowther, 2005:137). The extent to which caesarean protects against such adverse outcomes is not yet clear. Concerns about the benefits of caesarean are aggravated by knowledge that caesarean birth is associated with lower Apgar scores among higher multiple babies and respiratory problems in 36- to 38-week gestation twins (Dodd and Crowther, 2005:137). These conditions carry an increased risk of mortality as well as morbidity.

In an attempt to address these uncertainties about the preferred route of delivery for twins, an international multicentre randomised controlled trial (RCT) is being organised by the same research institute as hosted the late and unlamented Term Breech Trial (see section 2.5.2; Barrett, 2005). The research protocol suggests, however, that the findings of the Twin Birth Study (TBS) will not be available before the year 2011.

According to Newman (1998), the use of caesarean is even greater among the higher multiple pregnancies, at over 90 per cent. The rationale for this high caesarean rate is certainly not found in the research literature (Dodd and Crowther, 2005). The logic is that perinatal death is prevented by surgical intervention reducing the risk of the babies being in a poor condition as assessed by the Apgar scores at birth. It may be, though, that anxiety is a major factor in these cases, serving as an indication for a caesarean. The anxiety, however, is not just that of the parents but also the 'clinician's' (Penn and Ghaem-Maghami, 2001:7). As is becoming apparent in caesarean decision making, on such occasions, any research evidence plays only a relatively minor part in the caesarean decision.

5.2.2.2.5 INFECTIOUS CONDITIONS

Certain viral infectious in the mother may be transmitted to the baby during the birth process. For this reason, caesarean may sometimes be recommended as a means of bypassing the birth canal in order to reduce the risk of the baby developing a neonatal infection.

5.2.2.2.5.1 Herpes Simplex Virus (HSV) Neonatal herpes is a serious condition, in that it carries a mortality rate of 50–60 per cent (Marks et al, 1999). The baby is most likely to contract this infection if the woman's first infection with genital herpes happened less than six weeks before the birth. In these circumstances, there is a 40–60 per cent risk of the baby being infected. The most effective approach to the prevention of neonatal herpes is the combined treatment with antiviral drugs of both the women and her sexual partner (Barnabas et al, 2002). Marks and colleagues found that, were this woman to request a caesarean for her baby's sake, the more senior medical staff were significantly more likely to agree to it. Those medical staff in private practice would be similarly amenable. These researchers, though, conclude that only rarely does the relatively small risk of infecting the baby justify the risks of caesarean to the mother (Marks et al, 1999).

5.2.2.2.5.2 Human Immunodeficiency Virus (HIV) The most frequent route by which a child can become infected with HIV is from her mother during the birth process. This route may be known as mother to child transmission (MTCT) or vertical transmission. The proportion of babies thought to become infected in this way has been steadily declining since the possibility of vertical transmission was first recognised. It is now thought that between 15 and 35 per cent of HIV infected mothers transmit the virus to their babies (Newell, 2006). In developed countries where prophylactic antiretroviral therapy is available, elective caesarean can be provided and relatively safe alternatives to breast feeding exist, vertical transmission is able to be reduced to less than 2 per cent (ECS, 2005). On the other hand, the picture is less optimistic in countries where there is a lack of a clean water supply for reconstituting formula, where elective caesarean is seriously hazardous for the woman and antiretroviral therapy is the sole therapeutic agent.

The risks of caesarean for the woman have been addressed elsewhere (see Chapters 5 and 6). These risks, however, have been shown to be particularly grave, in terms of both maternal morbidity and mortality, for the woman who is infected with HIV (Miller, 1988; Semprini et al, 1995; Dathe et al, 1998). The risks include both the ordinarily relatively minor problems, such as pyrexia and anaemia, as well as more serious conditions such as wound infections, peritonitis, sepsis and pneumonia, possibly leading to death. Thus, it would appear that, yet again, the woman is accepting caesarean for the benefit of her baby, while putting her own health and even her life in jeopardy.

A relatively low-tech intervention has been introduced, which may reduce the need for elective caesarean by making vaginal birth safer for the baby of a woman with HIV. This intervention involves the disinfection of the woman's birth canal during labour by manual cleansing using microbicides. In this way, the likelihood of the baby making contact with the mother's infectious body fluids, such as cervical mucus and vaginal secretions, and contracting HIV is intended to be reduced (Wiysonge et al, 2005). A large RCT involving 6,964 women was undertaken in Malawi to investigate the effectiveness of this low-tech intervention (Biggar et al, 1996). The researchers found that there was no significant difference between the babies of the control and the experiment groups. If the membranes had been ruptured for more than 4 hours before the birth, though, the experiment group babies fared significantly better than the control group babies. In these circumstances, only 25 per cent of the babies in the experiment group contracted the virus, compared with 39 per cent in the control group. A faulty randomisation process, though, means that these findings may not be completely reliable. A systematic review by Wiysonge and colleagues concludes that evidence is lacking to support the use of this simple, low-cost and relatively woman-friendly intervention. They go on to plead for an authoritative RCT.

5.2.2.2.6 TOCOPHOBIA

Fear has traditionally been a close companion of childbirth. Such fear is entirely rational (Bewley and Cockburn, 2004). The nature or object of that fear, however, has changed over time. For seventeenth-century women, the 'frequent tragedies' that were the death of a mother (Marshall, 1983:114) caused women to prepare for labour as they would prepare themselves for dying (Mander, 2006b:131). More recently, as its likelihood has receded, fear of death has been replaced by other fears. Fear was the initiating problem, identified by Grantly Dick-Read (1933), in his triad leading, by way of tension, to labour pain. The object of the fear was not entirely clear, although he sought to address the woman's fear of the unknown through educational interventions.

Similarly, although tocophobia (sometimes known as tokophobia) has long been discussed, the precise object of the woman's fear has only recently been identified (Eriksson et al, 2006). For some women, the claim to tocophobia comprises a fear of pregnancy, as found in self-help websites. More usually, the woman's fear relates to the labour or the actual birth, which reflects the origins of the term, which are found in '*tocos*' or '*tokos*', the Greek word for childbirth. Again, though, the precise focus of the fear tends to remain unstated. The assumption may commonly be made that the labour pain is the reason, but other fears, such as loss of control, dread of hospitals, fear of self-exposure or reluctance to sever the bond with the fetus, may also feature.

In an attempt to classify 'tokophobia' for the first time, it was defined in terms of it being 'an unreasoning dread of childbirth' which is 'so intense that childbirth is avoided whenever possible' (Hofberg and Brockington, 2000:83). In the course of their qualitative study, these researchers identified women who had never been pregnant and who manifested 'primary tokophobia'. For these women, the pain of labour appears to be the focus of their fears, as an elective caesarean is presented as the solution to their phobic state. 'Secondary tokophobia' is said to be associated with a previous traumatising experience, such as an instrumental or operative birth.

Many of these women had convinced themselves that they and their babies would die. Hofberg and Brockington attribute tokophobia to psychiatric morbidity, such as depression or post traumatic stress disorder (PTSD) following sexual abuse. These researchers discuss the women's motivation for pregnancy, that is, their 'overwhelming desire to be a mother [which was] their *raison d'être*' (2000:83). In spite of having been able to overcome their fears sufficiently to conceive, some of the women still found it necessary to undergo a termination of pregnancy when the reality of childbearing faced them. Thus, these researchers demonstrate the 'unreasoning' nature and 'intensity' of these women's dread.

As with many health problems which begin as genuinely incapacitating, toco-phobia has become devalued. This is apparent in this term's use in the lay media (Williams, 2005). The risk-averse nature of western society is well recognised and this journalist also reports women's lack of confidence in their ability to become mothers. Her interviewee then observes 'people are so frightened of childbirth. What's it called, tocophobia? Well it's called that now! It didn't even exist before!'

The treatment for tocophobia, as mentioned already, has been recommended to be elective caesarean. It may even be that tocophobia has actually become recognised as an indication for caesarean. This form of therapy, and possibly the condition itself has been called into question by Swedish research. An obstetrician with a psychotherapeutic orientation undertook a series of consultations with 100 women with a 'fear of delivery', the majority of whom were seeking a caesarean (Sjögren, 1998). Following the psychological support offered to these women, more than half of those initially seeking a caesarean decided to opt for a vaginal birth. These women were found to be satisfied with their revised decision and enjoyed a birth experience as good as those women without a fear of childbirth. When Ryding and her colleagues (2003) undertook a similar but midwife-led study in another Swedish setting, the results were less encouraging. Although the women in the psychotherapeutic treatment group were happy with their care by the 'fear of childbirth team', their experience of birth was seriously negative, relative to the comparison group.

The use of tocophobia as a rationale for undertaking caesareans for which there is no other indication is raised as a source of concern by some authors (Leeman, 2005). Clearly, a morbid and incapacitating fear of childbirth is all too real for a number of women. That this diagnosis, though, may be used by both women and their attendants to justify unnecessary caesareans, is a possibility. The question of who should be 'blamed' for this sorry state has already been asked (Di Renzo, 2003). This astute commentator identifies, without naming it, the potential for an unholy alliance to arise. On one side of the alliance is the pregnant woman seeking to avoid 'nature's obligations'. On the other side, the ally is the 'condescending obstetrician [evading attending] a labour while gaining more income and at the same time giving his patient the illusion of happiness' (Di Renzo, 2003:217).

Clearly, the reality of tocophobia and the use or misuse to which this term is being put, are in urgent need of serious research attention.

5.2.2.3 Summary

This section has demonstrated the dynamic processes which influence the indications for performing a caesarean. I have shown how the indications for this operation have changed and are changing with a variety of factors, such as time, pathophysiology and technology, to name but a few. These changes mean that this major operation is now more likely to be performed when the indications are less marked or less severe than was previously the case. Additionally, certain other factors serve to further lower the threshold for the performance of a caesarean. These include, in the woman, the level of anxiety, or in the baby, size, degree of compromise, or number of babies. This bringing down of the caesarean threshold has been facilitated by a widespread perception of the increasing 'routineness', safety and ease of caesarean. Thus, this aspect of the dynamic nature of caesarean is influenced by public perceptions as well as by medical decision making.

This phenomenon may be an example of the 'push–pull' effect. This is when the movement of an object is brought about by the combined effect of two forces which, though diametrically opposed, may actually serve to enhance each other's efforts. So, while medical decisions tend to emphasise the ease, convenience and relative certainty of caesarean, they permit the public perception that this operation is 'pain free' and benefits baby and mother to pass unchallenged. Thus, the door to increasing the caesarean rate is being pushed open by one group and pulled open by the other. In section 5.2.2.2.6, I referred to an unholy alliance which serves to increase the number of caesareans for one particular indication. It may be that such an alliance acts to achieve the short-term aims of both groups, although it may be that only the medical profession benefits in the long term. It would appear, on the basis of this discussion, that the decision making remains in the domain of the medical practitioner.

5.3 Maternal choice/request/demand for caesarean

The word that is used to portray this phenomenon, of the woman actively seeking a caesarean, is really determined by the role and position of the person using it. Thus, 'choice' may be more accepting, whereas a 'demand' is clearly to be condemned. In the interests of moderation, I will opt for the middle way, by referring to 'requests'.

5.3.1 Perceptions and numbers

There is a widespread and possibly growing perception that the number of women choosing, requesting or demanding caesarean without any health problems to justify it is increasing. This perception of greater numbers is well known in the popular press (see Introduction and section 1.4.7) and is even reflected in the professional media (Arthur and Payne, 2005:17). Whether this perception is accurate is difficult to assess because of the complexity of the negotiations around the birth decision (please see next paragraph). It has been suggested that the number of requests for caesarean varies according to who you ask. Obstetricians are said to perceive a high rate of such requests, in contrast to the childbearing women (Anderson, 2006). Even if these perceptions of increasing requests are not correct and women's behaviour is not changing as much as thought, the number of column inches devoted to this possibility has escalated exponentially since 1985 (Wax et al, 2004:602).

The reality of any increase in the incidence of caesarean on request must depend to some extent on what is meant by 'request'. In birth decision making, as in any negotiations, there is an element of 'brinksmanship', when either party will seek to 'read' the position of the other and meet or address their perceived demands. The delicacy and complexity of these negotiations, some of which may not even have been explicit, emerges in the important study by Weaver and Statham (2005). As in the 'push–pull' analogy mentioned already (see section 5.2.2.3), one party may encounter less resistance than they had anticipated and, as a result, may become more enthusiastic in their determination. Alternatively, a person with a request in mind may be deterred from even articulating it by the appearance, demeanour or gender of the other. Such delicate balances and adjustments are impossible to identify by surveys and audits, so may pass unnoticed. For these reasons, the numbers of caesareans on request remains open to 'impressions' and 'interpretations'.

In spite of this proviso, attempts have been made to count the requests. A North American perspective suggests that caesarean on request constitutes between 4 per cent and 18 per cent of all caesareans (Wax et al, 2004). This figure is supposedly supported by a survey of England, Wales and Northern Ireland, which found that clinicians reported that an average of 7.3 per cent of caesareans were performed primarily because of maternal request (Thomas and Paranjothy, 2001:23). This average, though, conceals a variation which is said to range between 6.1 per cent in the north west of England and 8.4 per cent in the south east of England. Individual maternity units, however, were found to demonstrate an even wider range of between 2 per cent and 27 per cent of caesareans for maternal request. Interestingly, the figure that women in Scotland reported for being able to choose caesarean almost matched the figure mentioned by 'clinicians' in the remainder of the UK at 7 per cent (Graham et al, 1999).

5.3.2 *Ethics*

The first fundamentally important ethical principle which determines matters such as the availability of caesarean on request is the 'duty of care' (Melia, 2004). It must be recognised that judgements by health care personnel about care are all too often based on inadequate or incomplete knowledge. The decision to undertake an intervention like caesarean, without convincing indications and with even the slimmest risk of harm to mother or baby, violates that duty of care. That a risk exists is apparent (see Chapters 6 and 7) and has also been argued on the grounds that if it did not exist it would be necessary to offer caesarean 'to all women' (Bewley and Cockburn, 2004:187). On this basis, the ethical principle of non-maleficence becomes paramount, although some would suggest that the woman's autonomy surpasses it. This argument was addressed in the overused paper by Paterson-Brown

(1998), which concluded that caesarean should be available on request as long as the woman is fully informed. She bases this recommendation on her two assumptions, the first of which is that caesarean is 'a safe mode of delivery' (1998:463). Secondly and equally inappropriately, she assumes that being 'fully informed' (1998:462) is feasible, even when she herself admits that 'the evidence is incomplete' (1998:462).

5.3.3 Maternal mortality and morbidity

In spite of Paterson-Brown's assumptions, maternal mortality is indisputably higher in association with caesarean. The rates, however, are not static. The mortality rate for vaginal births in the UK hovers at around 17–20 deaths per million cases. As reported in the 'Confidential Enquiries', the mortality rate for elective caesarean was declining markedly until 1994–96 (Lewis, 1998). After this time the mortality rates for elective and emergency caesareans ceased to be presented separately. In the 1994–96 report, though, the mortality rate for elective caesareans, at 58.5 per million cases, was almost three times higher than for vaginal births. The mortality rate for emergency caesareans was falling, but more slowly than the rate for elective operations. In the 1994–96 report, the mortality rate for emergency caesareans, at 182.0 deaths per million cases, was more than three times higher than for elective operations. The overall picture of these rates, in the most recent (2000–02) report, is not markedly different, although the authors caution against reading too much into these figures (Lewis, 2004).

The unwillingness of health professionals to contemplate the possibility of the death of a mother emerged out of my own research (Mander, 2001b; 2001c). That such an argument could or should ever be used to enlighten or persuade a child-bearing woman is difficult to imagine. Thus, there remains the assumption, as expounded by Paterson-Brown (1998), that caesarean is the safe option for both the baby and the woman.

As well as the still taboo topic of maternal death, there is another form of morbidity which needs to be taken into account in this highly publicised debate. The role of the media should not be underestimated, especially when celebrities choose to give birth by caesarean performed on request. The effect of such media hype on women's deeply held anxieties about giving birth is to confirm in their minds that labour is inherently dangerous and caesarean is the way to avoid such dangers. In this way, as Bewley and Cockburn astutely observe, caesarean on request 'reinforces cultural apprehension' (2004:186)

5.3.4 Research

The lack of authoritative research evidence to demonstrate the relative benefits of caesarean as opposed to vaginal birth was noted by Paterson-Brown as long ago as 1998. On the basis of a brief search, I have found that this still applies at the time of writing. For this reason, it is necessary to use the existing research on mortality and morbidity (see section 5.3.3). Although it sounds implausible, the possibility of an RCT comparing elective caesarean with planned vaginal birth has been seriously discussed (Wax et al, 2004:612). More sensibly a midwife writer dismisses this possibility as 'very unlikely' (Anderson, 2006:35).

5.3.5 Choice

The crucial role of maternal choice has been the subject of virtually infinite rhetoric since it featured as one of the 'Three C's' in the Changing Childbirth Report (DoH, 1993). Along with control and continuity, choice was expected to convert maternity care into a woman-centred service. That these aims have not been achieved is generally, though sadly, recognised (Rothwell, 1996). In spite of its limited success at policy level, this rhetoric continues to be well rehearsed. Medical adherence to the woman's 'choice', though, bears little relation to the woman's autonomy and is seriously circumscribed by the dictum of non-maleficence (Bewley and Cockburn, 2004). As Paterson-Brown cynically yet accurately observes, freedom of choice only exists as long as it is the right choice (1998:463).

In the context of caesarean, the woman's choice is clear if it is the recommended form of treatment in the event of some form of maternal or fetal pathology. In such circumstances, in the UK, the woman has the right to decline caesarean (see section 5.5). The woman's right to refuse recommended treatment has been clearly established if her or her baby's condition arouses some concern. The situation in healthy circumstances is less clear, though. While the woman may refuse an intervention, is it possible for her to request an intervention when there is not a health problem to serve as an indication?

5.3.6 Rights

Women's rights to self-determination underpin many aspects of maternity care and may clarify choice issues. These rights are crucial to the woman's autonomy, but some distinction is necessary. As mentioned already, the woman's negative rights, that is her right to refuse an intervention, is clearly established, even if her health and her baby's is thought to be at risk. What is less clear, though, is whether there exist any positive rights for the woman to request an intervention in the absence of a health problem or other indication. Thus, a conflict develops between the woman's right to make autonomous decisions and the health worker's rights to practise according to accepted professional standards (Amu et al, 1998).

5.3.7 Professional issues

The roles of the two main disciplines or professions who are responsible for advising and attending the childbearing woman are clearly different. The differences are thrown into sharp relief by the issue of caesarean on request. The midwife claims to be the health professional who is 'with woman', and whose role is to support and facilitate healthy childbearing with an emphasis on 'normality'. It may even be that the midwife has a 'vested interest' in 'normal' childbearing, as it is the sum total of what she is able to offer (Bewley and Cockburn, 2004:186). The role of the midwife if a woman seeks to request a caesarean is less clear. On the one hand, the midwife should support the woman in whatever decision she chooses to make. On the other hand, the midwife may try to find out from the woman her reasons for seeking to avoid giving birth vaginally (Arthur and Payne, 2005).

The role of the obstetrician is certainly different. Bewley and Cockburn (2004: 186) reflect on the position of the conscientious medical practitioner and the implications of a request for caesarean in terms of the practitioner's and the service's resources. As these authors conclude, though, the history of obstetrics is firmly embedded in gynaecological surgery. One might even go as far as to state that surgery is the obstetrician's *raison d'être*. Thus, operations such as caesarean may be perceived as the obstetrician's unique selling point (USP). It is hard, to say the least, to imagine any discipline or occupational group attempting to limit the use of their USP.

The role of the medical practitioner is shown to be somewhat paradoxical by an observation by Barrett (2004:629). This is a group which has not traditionally been recognised for its encouragement of women's autonomy. It is now being noted, though, that this situation is changing. Regrettably, it has now been noticed that medical practitioners are now less concerned to reduce caesarean rates. The corollary of this development, for some inexplicable reason, is a mass movement 'towards supporting maternal choice for method of delivery' (Barrett, 2004:629).

5.3.8 Prophylaxis

Whereas I have been considering the issues relating to caesarean 'on request', some medical authorities refer to this phenomenon as 'prophylactic caesarean' (Wax et al, 2004; Paterson-Brown, 1998). The concept of prophylaxis is essentially about preventing some adverse or unwanted outcome, such as an infection or pain. The question which now needs to be addressed is against what does caesarean on request serve as prophylaxis? One possibility is that the answer to this question may be found in the uncertain beginnings and outcomes of labour (Bewley and Cockburn 2004:186). It may be that a woman may seek certainty in this aspect of her life, as in others. A more serious possibility is that the only outcome that can, with any degree of certainty, be avoided by caesarean on request is the spectre of emergency caesarean. It could be that this outcome, with its loss of maternal control and increased morbidity and mortality rates is what the 'requests' are actually seeking to avoid. The emergency caesarean has been linked already with certain interventive practices which form part of the cascade of intervention (see section 1.4.9). It may be, therefore, that it is these interventive practices in labour which are to be avoided by a prophylactic operation, in an effort to prevent or reduce the possibility of the unsatisfactory outcome.

Thus, although, this scenario may have been dubbed 'caesarean on demand' any demands are clearly being manipulated with a view to conforming with the medical agenda.

5.4 Other factors influencing the caesarean decision

Up to this point, a number of phenomena have been shown to influence the likelihood of the decision being made for the woman to undergo a caesarean. These phenomena have been shown to include private medical practice, the woman's relative degree of affluence, the woman's fear of vaginal birth and maternal request, as well as a range of health problems. In this section, I scrutinise certain less tangible factors which are likely to influence the caesarean decision.

5.4.1 The technological imperative

Because the caesarean comprises a surgical technique rather than a form of technology, it may be argued that there is no way the decision can be said to be driven by the technological imperative. It is necessary to consider carefully, though, whether this drive is in any way relevant to caesarean decision making. I would argue that technology is a fundamental building block of the medical model. This model derives from the separation of the functioning of the mind and the body and regarding the human body, in a Cartesian way, like a machine. In the event of a fault or illness, attention is needed to repair the fault. When considering maternity care from this reductionist point of view, the technological imperative would appear to be germane to the caesarean decision.

The Norwegian ethicist, Hofmann (2002) would not agree. He argues, from the moral high ground, that health care providers are entirely logical and objective in their decisions to use technology. There is apparently no attraction for this ethicist in the seductive nature of either the quick fix or the easy answer. To counter Hofmann's viewpoint, I would argue that there are a number of quite subjective factors which have influenced the decision to employ technology. It is by no means unknown for the availability of a technique to have influenced, or even determined, obstetric practice. One pertinent example would be the virtually universal practice of routine prophylactic episiotomy in the 1970s (Graham, 1997). Other examples would include equipment so basic as to be barely deserving of the label 'technology', such as the safety razor or the obstetric bed (Murphy-Black, 1990; Boenigk, 2006).

The likelihood of health care personnel being seduced by technology is blamed on 'the industrialisation of health care' (Barnard, 1999:440) together with the biomedical model. The consequences associated with such a seduction, Barnard maintains, are found in iatrogenic conditions. Rather than throwing the technological baby out with the bathwater, Barnard recommends that progress in health care should be achieved by using it more appropriately, together with 'scholarship, wisdom, research, human experience, art, science and spirituality' (1999:440). Thus, a range of higher order obligations would operate alongside technology.

5.4.2 Peer pressure in favour of caesareans

The medical profession is well known for offering effective mutual support to its members. Its cohesiveness emerges in any number of well-publicised cases. One particular *cause célèbre* is the case that became known by the name of the book about it, that is, the 'Savage Enquiry' (Savage, 1986). The precise issues involved in this case may never be entirely clear; the situation that was portrayed by the media, though, comprised a group of male obstetricians objecting to the woman-centred practice of their female colleague, Mrs Wendy Savage. While the incidents which instigated her suspension related to her reluctance to perform unnecessary caesareans, the conflict with her male colleagues was due to her unwillingness to follow the policies and practices to which they fervently adhered. Her penalty for not toeing the 'party' line was her suspension from practice. This eventually ended with her total exoneration in July 1986 (Pratten, 1990). One interpretation of this case is that the usual cohesive behaviour of the male obstetricians was expected to apply pressure to Savage to persuade her to bring her practice into line. Unfortunately, her medical brethren underestimated her ability to manipulate both the media and the public on her own behalf.

Thus, this case is an example of medical peer pressure being peculiarly ineffective. Another useful example features peer pressure being used effectively and, as Savage's protagonists would have wished, to maintain the medical *status quo*. In Canada, Enkin and his evidence-minded colleagues sought to encourage medical practitioners to perform fewer caesareans (Enkin, 1992). This encouragement involved providing information about the lack of research evidence to support the routine use of caesarean in a breech presentation or after a previous caesarean. While apparently accepting of the research evidence, the medical practitioners changed their practice only barely perceptibly (see section 2.7). Reflecting on the dismal failure of this introduction of evidence-based practice, Enkin considers that it is the local influences which determine medical practice decisions: 'Every day experiences and contacts, and the views and practices of respected colleagues in their community, are more powerful . . .' (1992:217) Enkin goes on to conclude that 'local peer pressure' is sufficiently strong to prevent physicians from changing their behaviour. This finding endorses the work of Tussing and Wojtowycz, who observed 'the strong effect of peer influence in the form of county and adjusted hospital rates' (1997:187). Again, the overpowering message between medical practitioners is to hold the line, which results in the inexorable rise in the caesarean rate.

5.4.3 Defensive obstetric practice

The fear of litigation is widely believed to be at least partly responsible for the increasing intervention rate in maternity care. This fear inevitably affects practice and increases the likelihood of decisions being made to undertake a caesarean (Churchill et al, 2006:53). The rationale is that if the medical practitioner has been seen to have 'done something' s/he is less likely to be sued, than if s/he waited for nature to take its course. The fact that this 'something', such as caesarean, may actually cause more problems, that is, it is iatrogenic, does not appear to feature in this Alice in Wonderland logic. Wagner examines this topsy-turvy rationale by asking the question 'How safe is [caesarean]?' (2000:1677). The answer, he argues, depends on who is answering the question. Wagner maintains that, in the absence of a caesarean, the medical practitioner considers her/himself to be taking the risk and adopting an untenable position. On the other hand, if a caesarean is performed, the evidence suggests that the risks are, unbeknown to her, to the health and life of the woman.

An authoritative mixed-method research project (Symon, 2000a; 2000b) supports Churchill and colleagues' contention that rising caesarean rates are linked to fear of litigation (2006). Symon's study shows the perception among both midwives and obstetricians that the increase in the number of caesareans is an example of defensive practice. Symon notes, paradoxically, that although Scotland has a higher caesarean rate than England (see section 4.3.1), perceptions of the effects of defensive practice are greater in England. It may be suggested that such a perception may serve as a deterrent to increasing caesareans, as it may engender reflection about to whom the benefits accrue.

The link between more general defensive practice and caesarean has been suggested as operating in two ways. First, the indirect effects of defensively using more investigations, such as continuous electronic fetal monitoring (CEFM), serve to increase the caesarean rate for suspected fetal compromise. Second, the decision to undertake an elective caesarean, to avoid a potentially risk-prone labour, would be a direct effect (Tussing and Wojtowycz, 1997).

The question needs to be asked about whether litigation, and the associated defensive obstetric practice, could be another transatlantic import. In countries such as the USA, where midwifery has long been weak to the point of barely existing, the caesarean rate has been higher than in countries where the midwifery presence is more firmly established (see Chapter 4). While caesarean rates escalate in health care systems which feature private practice, state financial support may not be provided to help to care for a baby born with a condition like cerebral palsy. Hence, if a baby is born affected, her parents have no choice but to take the obstetrician to court, if they are to fund the upbringing of a baby/child/person with disabilities. Thus, the vicious spiral of caesarean litigation and defensive practice is not only maintained, but actually escalates.

Whereas this vicious spiral manifests itself in countries with a high caesarean rate, reciprocally, the reverse applies in certain low-caesarean countries. In the Netherlands, for example, neglectful practitioners are disciplined, but compensation does not enter the equation. Instead, the health care system provides complete financial support for the childrearing costs. This removes any need to resort to litigation and forestalls any effects on midwifery and obstetric practice.

5.4.4 *Experience and personal opinion*

The role of personal experience should not be underestimated in the care decisions which health personnel make (Mander, 1992). A famous, or perhaps infamous, attempt was made in England to demonstrate the benefits of caesarean by showing the large proportion of obstetricians who would choose a caesarean for themselves or their female partners (Al-Mufti et al, 1996). The authors distributed postal questionnaires to 282 obstetric medical staff in NHS maternity units in London. Although the questionnaires were sent to consultant obstetricians, and senior training grades, no detail is provided of the proportions despatched or returned by each grade. The response rate was 73 per cent, which is high for a postal survey. Much media mileage has been made from the 31 per cent of the female respondents who stated that they would request an elective caesarean in the event of an 'uncomplicated singleton presentation at term'. This figure is significantly different from the male respondents of whom only 8 per cent would seek a caesarean for their partner. Although couched in terms of a question these practitioners' conclusion is that 'caesarean should be offered routinely to all pregnant women' (1996:544). The provenance of this survey arouses serious misgivings. This is partly due to the lack of detail about the sample, as some personnel who were eligible to be sent a questionnaire did not receive one (Robinson, 2002/03). The concerns are mainly due to the mode of publication. This survey was published in the form of a letter. In this way the authors bypassed the rigours of peer review and ensured that only minimal detail and data were able to be provided, while maximum publicity was obtained.

A similar survey in Scotland produced rather different findings, but has attracted infinitely less media attention. MacDonald and her colleagues (2002) sent questionnaires to all of the female obstetricians of registrar grade or above in Scotland. Of the 100 questionnaires distributed, 90 were returned completed. Seventy of these respondents (77.8 per cent) claimed that they would not choose a caesarean and 6.6 per cent were not sure. Of the 15.6 per cent of respondents (n=14) who stated that they would choose a caesarean, a large majority had no personal experience of childbearing. The proportion of the obstetricians who were mothers and who would choose a caesarean was small at 7 per cent. None of those who had ever given birth vaginally would seek an elective caesarean. That these data, which are distinctly unfavourable to caesarean, were collected in a country where caesarean rates are generally higher, must cast further serious doubt on the findings of Al-Mufti and his colleagues in London.

Another survey was undertaken in the north of England to find out how female midwives viewed the possibility of being able to choose a caesarean (Dickson and Willett, 1999). In this study, the response rate among the 135 practising midwives who were sampled was even higher than the medical surveys, at 100 per cent. The same hypothetical uncomplicated situation was presented and 95.5 per cent (n=129) of the midwives stated a preference for a vaginal birth. The authors contemplate the different experiences of the various professionals involved in maternity care and how this experience may influence their personal preferences and opinions.

Dickson and Willett emphasise the midwife's experience of caring for a new mother who is recovering from a caesarean and endeavouring to look after her baby. This experience is in stark contrast to the experience of the obstetrician, who is unlikely to encounter the immediate aftermath of the caesarean. The obstetrician's opinion and personal preference is likely to be based on her/his experience of medicalised labours which have become prolonged, or fetal compromise has been identified. The obstetrician's experience of providing care in an uncomplicated labour is, for obvious reasons, limited. The same may apply to their expertise in such a labour. Dickson and Willett conclude that childbearing women should be made aware of the overwhelming preference among midwives for vaginal birth. It may be argued that women should also be informed of the basis of the medical opinions and preferences which are all too often presented as expert, or even scientific, knowledge.

5.4.5 The partner's influence

In the UK the vast majority of fathers are present during the labour and at the birth (MacMillan, 1994; RCM, 1995). Research into why they are there and any effects associated with their presence are sadly lacking. What has been shown, both anecdotally and through research, is that the father encounters difficulty in coping with the uncertainties which he inevitably faces, even in a labour which at least begins by being uncomplicated (Mander, 2004a). The uncertainties with which the father has difficulty coping are manifold. They include uncertainty about, first, the outcome of the labour in terms of the health of the woman and the baby. Second, are the uncertainties relating to the duration of the labour, which appear to be challenging. The third and greatest uncertainties have been shown to be those arising out of the father's misgivings about his partner's labour pain. These misgivings relate not only to the severity of the pain, but also to the father's feelings of disappointment about his inability to remedy his partner's pain.

Through the medicalisation of childbearing, the obstetrician has sought to resolve both his and the father's uncertainties about the unknown outcome, the duration and the pain of labour. The resolution of these uncertainties may also be welcomed by some women (see section 4.3.4). The changes contributing to medicalisation, with the intention of ensuring better outcomes, have featured greater surveillance. This applies both to the maternal condition, in the form of observing progress in labour, and also to the fetal condition, through the increased use of continuous electronic fetal monitoring (CEFM). The duration of labour has been manipulated through the use of the partograph; this documentation (see section 4.1.1) is difficult to separate from the interventions to accelerate labour, using the principles of active management, which it demands. Through the cascade of intervention, there emerges an increased likelihood of other procedures to hasten and terminate the labour, such as the caesarean operation for 'failure to progress'. Thus, a link may begin to emerge between the father's presence and the likelihood of the caesarean operation.

5.5 Non-consensual caesarean

Up to this point in this chapter, the focus of caesarean decision making has quite correctly been on the balance of how the decision is made between the woman and her health care providers. It is now necessary to move into those areas in which the woman may be even less involved in the caesarean decision. The first of these is those situations in which a caesarean may be performed not only without the agreement or consent of the childbearing woman, but actually contrary to her expressed wishes. In such circumstances the operation may, alternatively, be entitled court-ordered or enforced.

Prior to 1997, there were a number of these cases in England (Scott, 2000). Because Scotland has a different legal system, there has always been less chance of such occurrences there (Wilkinson and Norrie, 1993). The English cases appear to have been complicated by the tendency of the medical and legal professionals to be something less than stringent in their observance of the legal requirements (Burrows, 2001). In 1992, this tendency appeared in the case of Mrs S, a woman with deeply held religious beliefs (Hewson, 1994; Cahill, 1999). In an earlier pregnancy, she had been threatened with a stillborn or damaged baby if she did not agree to a caesarean. Her faith convinced her that it was not necessary and, after a two-day labour, she gave birth vaginally to a baby in a good condition. Thus, in her next pregnancy, she was disinclined to believe similar threats when she was found to have a transverse lie. The court hearing at which the caesarean decision was made involved neither Mrs S nor her representative, as is legally required. The Leading Counsel cited the American situation as evidence to support the need for the caesarean. This is a further travesty of justice, as the American legal system, unlike the English one, grants the fetus the rights of an individual. In English law the fetus has no personal rights until, at birth, s/he becomes an individual human being with the same rights as any other.

Some years later in 1996, a different woman, known as Ms S, was diagnosed with severe pre-eclampsia at 36 weeks' gestation (Caufield, 1999). Because Ms S sought an uncomplicated birth, her general practitioner was unable to persuade her to be admitted to a maternity unit with a view to expediting the birth. The practice social worker interviewed Ms S and made an application for admission to a psychiatric unit under Section 2 of the Mental Health Act of 1983 (Cahill, 1999). Soon after her admission to the psychiatric unit, Ms S was transferred to a maternity hospital even though there was no sign of labour. The hospital's lawyers applied to treat Ms S without her consent and the judge, Mrs Justice Hogg, who had been led to believe that she was in advanced labour, agreed the order. On this basis, without Ms S's consent and with no physical resistance, a caesarean was performed.

Subsequently Ms S applied for a judicial review to revisit the decision that she should have a caesarean against her will. In 1998 the Court of Appeal found that her treatment had been unlawful. The 'irregularities' related, first, to Ms S's admission to the psychiatric unit on the grounds of non-existent depression (Cahill, 1999). Second, her subsequent transfer to the maternity unit contravened mental health legislation. Third, Mrs Justice Hogg was led to believe that Ms S was in prolonged labour, when labour had not actually begun. The Court of Appeal's verdict was derived from the view that a pregnant woman is competent to make decisions about her treatment and her baby's. Interventions may not be performed unless the woman gives her consent even if there are risks to her and/or her baby's health. Thus, the law of consent applies during childbearing, just as much as it does at other times.

This verdict contradicts the widely held assumption that if a woman does not accept the guidance of her medical adviser, she must, by definition, be incompetent. This would make her unable to either give or withhold consent to treatment. Although she doesn't actually use the word, Cahill (1999) seems to regard the non-consensual caesarean as another example of 'fetocentric' care (Mander, 2004a:43). She contrasts the rhetoric of woman-centred care with the reality of interventions which are supposedly in the interests of the fetus. Non-consensual caesareans are a superb example of such a contrast. While the benefits to the fetus may be less than clear, the risks to the woman are well recognised. Thus, the balance between the welfare of the woman and the welfare of her baby appears to have swung too far in the direction of benefiting the baby. In this way, the medical interest in the fetus is seen to, not only disempower the woman, but also to jeopardise her health.

That the non-consensual caesarean may be another North American import emerges from the work of Harris (2001). She reports how this form of surgery appears to have become a growth industry in the USA. Of particular concern is the background of the women who have been subjected to this intervention which, in the UK, would legally constitute an assault. An overwhelming majority of the women (80 per cent) were 'African-American, African or Asian' (2001:95). Fifty per cent of the women were unsupported, and in more than one quarter (27 per cent) the woman's first language was other than English. Harris correctly goes on to articulate her suspicions that this group of relatively deprived women are vulnerable to this misplaced medico-legal intervention. Of course, these suspicions have been vehemently denied by those in favour by claiming the welfare of the fetus.

It may be that, as suggested already, non-consensual caesareans represent the at times far too cosy relationship between lawyers and medical practitioners. Such a relationship has been examined in terms of the 'maternal–fetal conflict' (Scott 2000:407). This legal fabrication bears a close resemblance to the medical assumption on which some non-consensual caesarean decisions are based and which may be typical of male-dominated professions who practise with women clients, in that it represents a supremely arrogant attitude. These practitioners assume that they, through their professional expertise, invariably carry a greater interest in the welfare of the baby than the mother does. While such attitudes may serve to perpetuate these professions' input into childbearing and childrearing, their basis is increasingly under attack.

The decision making in these examples of non-consensual caesarean is clearly to be deprecated. These decisions have been based on a paternalistic approach by the medical personnel, which has been closely linked with an arrogant assumption of maternal incompetence. The physiological condition of the baby was the prime, perhaps the only, consideration. Thus, this example is obviously the most blatantly extreme example of the caesarean decision not only being removed from the childbearing woman, but being taken and implemented in contradiction to her expressed refusal of the operation.

5.6 Higher order decisions

As mentioned already in section 1.1, the term and hence the origins of the caesarean operation are thought to derive from Roman legislation in the form of the *lex regia* or royal law. While the reason for this legislation is not entirely clear, the fact remains that an attempt was being required to remove the baby from a woman who was probably dead. The extent to which governmental and other high-level agencies have continued to exert an influence is a matter of some interest in view of the implications for the position of women and their health.

Another, possibly historical, influence on the obstetrician's caesarean decision was the Christian church. The impact of the Roman Catholic church on obstetricians in the nineteenth century was immense (Ryan, 2002). The church encouraged the rapidly developing caesarean operation, with the intention of saving the soul, and hopefully the life, of the baby. The alternative intervention, in the event of a woman's rachitic or 'rickety' pelvis causing obstructed labour, was a destructive operation (see section 1.2.4) and the removal of what remained of the baby. Such taking of innocent life, however, was deplored by church members. Thus, the church welcomed the caesarean because both of the 'patients' might survive (2002:462). The reality of this survival, though, was quite a different matter. While the more skilful surgeons might have been better able to boast a good survival rate, until at least the middle of the nineteenth century there were others whose practice was somewhat different. For this reason, many obstetricians were less than comfortable with the church's encouragement of caesarean. Ryan analyses the debate between obstetricians, and between obstetricians and theologians and the effect of changing ideas about the origin of human life. Ryan also draws attention to the unsurprising lack of involvement of women in these mighty deliberations.

The extent to which the church is still influential in encouraging caesareans is difficult to assess. Churchill (2003:48), however, maintains that this influence is still alive and well. This effect relates to the convenience of performing a sterilisation operation at the same time as a caesarean. The convenience of such surgery is likely to contribute to the high caesarean rates in Roman Catholic countries, such as Brazil (see section 4.2.3).

Although they are not a religious influence as understood by western people, the cosmic influences over a person's life are crucial in Chinese communities. These influences are largely determined by the hour, the day and the year of the birth, all of which may be controlled by an appropriately timed caesarean (Lo, 2003). For these reasons, Lo maintains, in mainland China caesareans are increasingly sought on the sixth day and the eighth day of the month because these numbers are associated with prosperity and wealth respectively.

Though obviously not a governmental body, the World Health Organisation (WHO) has clearly attempted to influence medical practice via governmental pressure to reduce the caesarean rate (see section 4.1.1). Thus, this is an example which demonstrates a directly opposing intention.

Although there may no longer be any specific high-level decisions to facilitate caesareans, it may be suggested that there are any number of government-level policies which serve to, perhaps inadvertently, increase the likelihood of more caesareans being performed. Some of these policies have been identified in the context of international comparisons (see section 4.3.5). Examples of such policy decisions would include the encouragement of private medical practice in countries such as Brazil and Greece. Further, certain governments have implemented policy decisions to limit the activities of midwives or to reduce the numbers being educated. This happened in the USA in the first half of the twentieth century (Jackson and Mander, 1995) and happened in China in 1993 (Cheung et al, 2005a). In both countries the lack of midwives was associated with reduced support for the woman in labour and an increase in the number of operative births (Hodnett et al, 2003).

An important example of a number of government-level decisions combining to increase, perhaps unexpectedly, the caesarean rate is found in the People's Republic of China (see section 4.2.2; Cheung et al, 2005a). The more infamous of these Chinese government decisions is the one child policy. Officially codified in 1979, the 'one child one family policy' (Doherty et al, 2001), established a system of rules and regulations governing the approved size of families in mainland China. These regulations included rewards for those who obeyed them, such as free maternity care. More disconcertingly, though, severe penalties were introduced and applied to couples who disobeyed the policy. The severity of these penalties is quoted by Doherty and colleagues (2001:746) as being in excess of one year's earnings. As with many aspects of life in China, the extent to which this policy is enforced varies, both according to place and with time. It should come as no surprise that in a country where medical care is as highly valued as it is in China, women seek caesareans in the hope of ensuring that there is no problem with their 'one child':

> 'I wanted to have a [caesarean]. The doctor did not think there was any clinical indication for it and refused . . . I argued with her. Then I reminded her that it seems I have the right to choose'.
>
> (Cheung et al, 2005b:36)

The popularity of the operation in China has resulted in a caesarean rate of 100 per cent in some areas, a development which may well have been aggravated by the steady demise of the midwifery profession there.

A less infamous example of intervention by a government somewhat closer to home is found in the Peel Report (DHSS, 1970). In a health care environment comprising a declining birth rate and an increasing maternity bed provision, the medical establishment sought to entrench its power base. The Peel Report did this by recommending 100 per cent hospital confinement. Other government reports had been produced earlier with slightly less extreme recommendations, but Peel was the most authoritative and most drastic. The rationale given in the report was that the greater safety conferred by hospital birth justified this recommendation. Also that all mothers should be able to 'benefit from the facilities available in hospital' (1970:24). The power base provided by Peel permitted the medical fraternity to embark on the obstetric excesses of active management which were characteristic of childbearing in the 1970s. The link between intervention in labour and caesarean has been established, resulting in the beginning of the escalation in caesarean rates (see section 1.3).

Thus, it is apparent that the decisions which increase the likelihood of a caesarean being performed are not only those that happen at a clinical level. The decisions made at the highest levels also influence the woman's birthing experience.

5.7 Conclusion

In this chapter I have shown the dynamic nature of caesarean decision making. This dynamic process is affected by a range of social and other phenomena. In spite of the more 'absolute' indications being widely regarded as non-negotiable, it is clear that the thresholds for the caesarean operation, like those which are performed for relative indications, are being changed. Tocophobia and caesarean on request/demand are examples of how the threshold to a caesarean being performed has been lowered. The technological and professional influences on the caesarean decision also need to be taken into consideration. Further, it is necessary to bear in mind the possibility of the caesarean being undertaken against the woman's wishes or following decisions relating to government policy or political factors.

Thus, it has become apparent in this chapter that, in a number of ways, the woman's input into the caesarean decision has changed. It has been shown that, in spite of media and other publicity suggesting the opposite, the woman's choice has been minimised or has even been quite blatantly overruled.

6 The immediate implications of caesarean

It may be because of the caesarean's ever increasing familiarity, that its ease, convenience and safety tend to be taken for granted. In this chapter, I begin to focus on some of the implications of the caesarean operation for the woman and her baby. I organise these ideas chronologically in the order in which the effects may manifest themselves. Thus, it is appropriate to consider the more immediate and shorter-term implications first. Eventually emerging out of this analysis there will be one major concept; this is that it is possible, as well as benefits, for harm to ensue after this intervention or treatment. Thus, I argue that caesarean may constitute a form of iatrogenesis. A discussion of what is meant by iatrogenesis and whether and to what extent it is relevant in this context will conclude this chapter.

6.1 The implications for the woman

There is a general assumption that caesarean is 'the easy way to have a baby', as Clement graphically demonstrates (1995:26). This research shows that even some medical personnel may tend to minimise the less positive aspects of the woman's experience of caesarean. It should not be surprising, therefore, that women and other people who have not previously undergone a caesarean may be quite ignorant of the reality of this experience:

> [Afterwards] I was aware of the most awful pain in my stomach, and couldn't understand why. I wondered if something has gone terribly wrong. I honestly hadn't realized I would be in pain!
>
> (Clement 1995:28)

In view of such a profound level of ignorance, it would not be surprising if, when offered a caesarean, some women feel at least a momentary feeling of relief that they do not have to endure, or endure any further, labour pain. In my experience, the woman will be persuaded of the necessity for a caesarean if such an offer is couched in terms of a reminder of the challenges of her labour so far, such as: 'You've been in labour now for so many hours; you must really be getting very tired . . .'

It is well nigh impossible, in my observation, for a woman who has been in labour for ten or twelve hours, having missed a night's sleep, to deny that she is tired. The woman's momentary relief at the proposal of a caesarean, though, is likely to be quickly supplanted by other feelings, concerns and thoughts of possible hazards. I address these hazards here, in order of their possible occurrence.

6.1.1 During surgery

Being a birth, the caesarean is ordinarily a happy event. For this reason, the potential for risks, which are inherent in any form of surgery, tend to be disregarded. The possible implications of fasting and of the introduction or induction of the anaesthetic are not being discussed here because they have already been addressed in sections 3.3.1.2. and 3.3.1.6.

6.1.1.1 Haemorrhage

Severe bleeding, which is likely to be uterine in origin, may occur during or after the caesarean operation. At the time of the operation, haemorrhage may be due to, first, abnormal development of the placenta which takes the form of, for example, placenta accreta (see section 7.1.5.1.1). Alternatively, haemorrhage may be due to trauma, to blood clotting disorders or to failure of the uterus to contract effectively (Bolbos and Sindos, 2005). There is general agreement that abnormal placental development is the most frequent cause of haemorrhage during caesarean operations (Baskett, 2003). While a small blood loss is probably unavoidable, the healthy woman's body is well able to cope with the loss of such an amount. A serious or 'massive' haemorrhage, though, is ordinarily defined as comprising a blood loss of one litre or more; this occurs in 7.3 per cent of caesarean operations (Jackson and Paterson-Brown, 2001).

Serious haemorrhage during caesarean is 'becoming more common', supposedly due to women giving birth at an older age, which may be associated with multiple pregnancy (Hall, 2004:87). Other reasons for the greater likelihood of haemorrhage, according to Hall, relate to women with chronic health problems embarking on childbearing, or to placental maldevelopment secondary to caesarean (see section 7.1.5). The continuing significance of 'catastrophic haemorrhage' as a cause of maternal mortality is demonstrated by Hall's chapter in the Confidential Enquiries into Maternal Deaths (2004:92).

In the event of haemorrhage occurring during the caesarean, the first line of treatment is conservative; that is, interventions such as oxytocic drugs are administered to control the bleeding. The limited success of this approach is evident from the plethora of other techniques which have been developed to minimise the uterine haemorrhage (Kwee et al, 2006; Bolbos and Sindos, 2005; Baskett, 2003). The ultimate intervention, though, is to surgically take out the source of the bleeding, that is, the removal of the woman's uterus by hysterectomy. The frequency with which it is necessary to resort to this ultimate surgical remedy is a reflection of the risks involved in caesarean. In the Netherlands, Kwee and colleagues (2006) found that hysterectomy was undertaken in 3.3 women per 10,000 births, whereas in Canada Baskett found that the equivalent rate was 5.3 (2003). Although the rate was lower in the Dutch series, the hysterectomy appears to have been less successful in saving the woman's life, as there were two maternal deaths (4 per cent, n=48). In the Canadian series, however, the higher removal rate was associated with no maternal loss of life.

6.1.1.2 Intra-operative awareness

The significance of 'awareness' as a seriously disabling experience, associated with caesarean under general anaesthesia, is only now beginning to be recognised (Osterman et al, 2001). Its impact was impressed on me when I was a very new midwife, by an encounter with a young woman who had just given birth by an emergency caesarean. She told me in great and accurate detail of her experience of having been aware of her heavy blood loss during the operation and the dramatic effect of this haemorrhage on the staff in the operating theatre. Her unimaginable anxiety was aggravated by her knowledge that, during her own birth by a caesarean twenty years earlier, her own mother had died due to an uncontrollable haemorrhage.

That this problem is now taken more seriously may be due to the relative infrequency of caesarean under general anaesthesia. The alternative explanation is the realisation of the existence of post traumatic stress disorder (PTSD) which may be caused by awareness. The problem of awareness is examined in greater detail in section 3.3.1.6.

6.1.1.3 The partner's presence

The presence of the partner at the birth is generally welcomed, or at least accepted. If the woman gives birth by caesarean under general anaesthesia, however, the staff may be inclined to veto his presence. It may be argued that this is the situation in which his presence in the operating theatre may be most important to the woman. This is because the partner's presence would mean that at least the father would be 'awake' to witness and welcome the baby. Probably equally importantly, he would be able later, to share with the mother a complete account (Hillan, 2000:72). In section 3.3.3 this problem is addressed in full.

6.1.1.4 Adverse incidents

As in any sphere of human activity, unpredictable events occur. Such events may be adverse and occasionally happen, in spite of training and checking systems, in the operating theatre. These events may include lack of communication or equipment failures (Lingard et al, 2004). These events also include those highly publicised incidents involving impostors posing as qualified personnel (Nuland, 2004).

6.1.1.5 Urinary catheterisation

The insertion of an indwelling catheter into the urinary bladder is one of those routine interventions which have become so standard in the preparation for a caesarean that 92.8 per cent of operators require it (NICE, 2004:55). As with so many routines, it is undertaken almost unthinkingly by staff, especially in emergency situations where time is of the essence. The rationale relates, first, to the bladder's close proximity and adherence to the lower segment of the uterus, where the incision is ordinarily made. An empty bladder is thought to be less likely to either get in the way or be damaged during surgery. This is a particular risk if regional anaesthesia is being used in view of the large fluid volumes infused together with the effect of the anaesthesia on bladder function. Second, women are usually informed that the catheter will remove the need for painful contortions to use bed pans for voiding in the early postoperative hours. Research into catheterisation during caesarean has focused on the risks of postoperative urinary retention (Page et al, 2003). Such changes in bladder function, though, may follow either a caesarean or an instrumental vaginal birth. Page and colleagues also discuss the effects on bladder function of different analgesic or anaesthetic medications.

An issue which does not appear to have been subjected to research scrutiny is the woman's reaction to this invasive procedure. It is my experience that some women find the presence of the indwelling catheter unpleasant to the point of being uncomfortable. Some women, because they have not been told how the catheter is held in position, become anxious about the pain of it being removed. The invasion by the catheter of the woman's bodily integrity is an issue which tends not to be discussed. Another potentially disconcerting aspect of this intervention is the way in which the catheter coverts the woman's ordinarily private urinary function into an all too 'public' matter (Ettinger, 2001). It may be that male obstetricians are not aware that, for women, urinating is usually a solitary and invariably an unseen activity.

6.1.2 *The early postoperative experience*

The postoperative care of the woman who has had a caesarean differs markedly from the care of a person who has undergone any other form of major abdominal surgery. Ordinarily, postoperative care comprises strict limitations on the activities of the recuperating 'patient'. In the event of a caesarean, however, the woman is not only not allowed such rest, but she is actively required to provide all care for her baby or babies.

6.1.2.1 Pain control

It is a basic tenet of pain management that 'Pain is what the person feeling it says it is', and this applies as much to post-caesarean pain as to any other. It is hardly surprising, therefore, that Clement (1995) identified a wide variation in women's experiences of post-caesarean pain. Whereas some women compared their pain favourably with that of women who had had a vaginal birth others, as mentioned above (please see section 6.1), fared less well:

> My first feeling was absolute shock that anything could be so painful. I suppose I had vaguely thought that caesareans were a less painful form of childbirth. It hurt me to cough, laugh, or even move slightly. Everything seemed a dreadful effort. I felt totally incapacitated.
>
> (1995:69/70)

In spite of the wealth of research literature on caesarean in general, the woman's experience of post-caesarean pain has not attracted recent research attention. This deficit, however, is to be corrected (Pearce and Dodd, 2004). The focus of recent research has been on the technical aspects, rather than on the woman's experience of and satisfaction with pain control. Such research has shown the benefits of intrathecal opioids and patient controlled analgesia, although both carry the risks of pruritis (itching) as well as nausea and vomiting. Wound infiltration with local anaesthetic has been evaluated experimentally, but its effectiveness is still not certain.

Because of the lack of recent woman-oriented research, it is necessary to draw on midwifery research which, although ground-breaking at the time, was undertaken more than a decade ago. The research to which I refer was that undertaken by Hillan and involved 100 women and a multiplicity of data collection methods. She found that the women experienced great difficulty in coping postnatally with 'the physical and psychological impact of major surgery, which may have occurred on top of a long and exhausting labour' (1992a:160). The women's wound pain was a major problem at this time. The women found that their hard time was compounded by their perception that 'the midwives were unaware of the difficulties [the women] had . . . in coping with the "aftermath" of this method of delivery' (1992a:168). While the women were still in hospital, a majority of them (68 per cent) were having trouble caring for the baby. These troubles related to activities ordinarily as simple as lifting and handling the baby, or moving into and out of bed or finding a comfortable position to adopt for feeding the baby.

Paradoxically, the anecdotal and research-based reality of experiencing the 'aftermath' of caesarean section appears to contrast markedly with the optimistic aims articulated by medical practitioners (OAA/AAGBI, 2005). This sorry situation is illuminated to some extent by nursing research into the decision making around the administration of analgesic medication (Willson, 2000). An ethnographic multiple-case study was undertaken in an English orthopaedic unit to study the rationale behind nurses' administration of pain relieving drugs. Willson found that certain organisational factors influenced the nurses' decisions. These included shift patterns and the impact of the multidisciplinary team. She also identified a widespread and continuing anxiety about the administration of opioid analgesics. This latter anxiety is particularly likely to feature among midwives in view of both the woman and the baby being vulnerable to the adverse effects of opioids. While nursing research is by no means automatically applicable to midwifery, I consider that these findings may be relevant in this context. Willson's findings clearly support the widespread anecdotal evidence of the persistence of Hillan's finding that post-caesarean pain control falls far short of being ideal or even adequate.

One exception to this observation that research is lacking is found in the work of Jakobi and colleagues (2002). These researchers examined the effectiveness of analgesic non-steroidal anti-inflammatory (NSAIDs) administered either on demand or three hourly on the first day post caresarean. Jakobi's group found that the 'on demand' mothers sought pain control in smaller quantities and less frequently. Perhaps unsurprisingly they reported higher pain scores and lower satisfaction with their pain control.

I have shown the limited research attention given to post-caesarean pain control. What little attention there is, though, has, probably appropriately, focused on wound pain. This means that the other forms of pain to which this new mother is particularly vulnerable appear to have been completely ignored. These other sources of pain include afterpains, intestinal wind pain and possibly perineal/haemorrhoidal pain.

The importance of effective pain control in the early days after a caesarean cannot be over-emphasised. The significance of controlling this new mother's pain relates not only to her feelings about herself; it also relates to her ability to provide care and nourishment for her baby, to her ability to mobilise in order to prevent other longer-term complications from arising and to resume some degree of normal functioning.

6.1.2.2 The hospital stay

If a woman who has a vaginal birth has chosen to go to a maternity unit to give birth, she and her baby may well be able to return home about six hours later. For the woman who has a caesarean, though, the situation is somewhat different. The NICE Guidelines (2004:14) recommend that the duration of the average stay is of three to four days, although the evidence base of this recommendation is unclear. These Guidelines go on to advocate that after caesarean a woman with no complications may be offered discharge from 24 hours after the birth; the rationale being that such early discharge is not linked to readmission for either mother or baby. This recommendation assumes that 'follow up at home' will be available. The nature of the 'follow up' is not specified, but it may comprise the care and support provided by the community midwife. Whether midwifery services will be able to continue to provide such a high level of support is not certain. It may be that a woman who has an elective caesarean is able to organise herself and those close to her in advance of the operation to ensure that her transfer home happens smoothly. Arrangements for domestic duties may also be pre-organised. The experience of the woman who has undergone an emergency caesarean, perhaps under general anaesthesia, would be totally different. Her physical and emotional recovery from her labour, her caesarean and her general anaesthetic would make it difficult for her to resume anything approaching her usual activities. Thus, the possibility of such an early transfer home for this woman would be fraught with problems.

The room in which the woman is accommodated while in the maternity unit will vary according to her condition and circumstances and according to the other demands, for example, for a single room. It is my experience that when caesareans were performed less frequently, it was easy to ensure that each woman returned postoperatively to her own single room; but with the increasing caesarean rate, this is no longer the case. Clement (1995) found that for some women a single room was important: 'I could be alone with my husband to sort my feelings out in private' (1995:66). For others it would have been welcome: 'I hardly got any sleep . . . When my baby was quiet it was someone else's baby crying' (1995:66). On the other hand, some women appreciated being in a larger room: 'The sharing of all our problems helped enormously, as nothing seems as bad when you can talk about it' (1995:66).

The time period spent in the maternity unit carries with it a number of risks. Some of these are largely physical, such as hospital acquired infection and thromboembolic conditions (please see section 6.1.3.2). There are, though, other less tangible risks. One of these is anxiety, which includes concerns that the woman may have difficulty recognising herself, let alone articulating to virtual strangers. For example, she may be anxious about how her separation from her existing child(ren) will affect her relationship with them. If the woman has any doubts about her partner, she may be worried about the state of the house, how well he is caring for any other children, perhaps what he is doing when not visiting her and with whom he is doing it. Although the woman in the maternity unit is likely to be busy with her new baby and her self-care, she may still feel isolated from her network of support. Such supports don't need to be human, as I learned from a woman who had had an emergency caesarean and whose overriding concern was whether her German shepherd dog was being fed, watered and walked correctly.

While in the maternity unit, especially if her caesarean was an emergency operation, she may feel frustrated that she is not able to implement all the plans which she had made for her return home with her new baby. Perhaps the most serious threat, though, is the threat to her confidence. This may arise from seeing staff dexterously handling the baby who she is barely able to lift. Alternatively, her loss of confidence may be due to seeing another mother feeding her baby full of formula, when her own supply of breast milk has yet to become established. Such anxieties and threats would not apply to a woman who went home at six hours after the birth, but because a woman who has had a caesarean usually stays for three to four days, they may develop into serious issues.

Thus, for some women, especially if it was unexpected, the stay in hospital may not be their happiest memory.

6.1.2.3 Eating and drinking

Policies relating to diet in labour have recently undergone a U-turn (see section 3.3.1.2). In the same way, ideas about the woman eating and drinking after a caesarean have also been turned around. The traditional practice of vetoing any oral intake until 'bowel sounds' could be heard was based on the twin fears of paralytic ileus and post anaesthetic vomiting (see section 6.1.3.3). A systematic review of the huge variations in post-caesarean dietary protocols concludes that they are certainly not based on research evidence (Mangesi and Hofmeyr, 2002). The reviewers go on to mention the 'discomfort' caused to women by the enforcement of such protocols, which is likely to be aggravated if the woman has previously been denied food and fluids during labour. On the basis of their incomplete systematic review, Mangesi and Hofmeyr report that there is no evidence base to support the withholding of oral fluids or food after a caesarean.

6.1.2.4 Baby care

As mentioned already, it is ordinarily the woman's responsibility to care for her healthy new baby while in the maternity unit. For reasons of security, removing the baby from the mother's care is not encouraged; but even though many maternity units no longer have a 'nursery', practice may vary. The availability of staff to help the woman with basic tasks such as nappy changing and positioning the baby for feeding may also vary according to the pressure of work. The support which midwifery staff provide is intended to prioritise breastfeeding, so the woman should be able to find assistance from those much needed extra pairs of hands in the early hours and days (Baston, 2005).

6.1.2.5 Support

In maternity care, it may be difficult to identify the boundaries between helping, teaching and supporting the new mother. As well as the practicalities, though, psychosocial support should ensure that the mother is encouraged to take all the decisions which an autonomous individual ordinarily takes. The educational aspects of support, however, become more significant for the woman who has undergone a caesarean, in view of the limited attention to this topic in childbirth education.

The care which is provided after a caesarean may be more fragmented than another mother's care because of the longer duration of stay in the maternity unit. The likelihood of such fragmented care providing effective support is difficult to assess. This fragmentation, however, may be further accentuated by the necessary input of other practitioners, such as physiotherapists, neonatal staff and medical personnel. A further threat to continuity of care and carer emerges in the work of Baxter and MacFarlane (2005). In response to adverse feedback from mothers, two new grades of staff were introduced to care for women following a caesarean. One group was registered general nurses, who were employed to meet the woman's postoperative needs. The other group was nursery nurses, who were employed to help the woman with baby care. The midwives were intended to practise specifically midwifery care. The researchers collected data by sending postal questionnaires to women who had had caesareans before and after the new staffing arrangements. The comparison of the 'before' and 'after' groups was based on the woman's recollection of, for example, having her wound checked. The researchers maintain that care was improved by this reorganisation of staff. They ignore the possibility of the Hawthorne effect and that members of the 'before' group obviously needed a better memory to recall events which, by definition, must have been more distant in time. Further, to those of us who have been working in health care for a lengthy period, the dismal spectre of organising care by task allocation would appear to be re-emerging.

6.1.3 Potentially serious health problems

There is a number of complications to which the woman is particularly vulnerable after a caesarean. These problems may be associated with her longer hospital stay, with this woman's relative immobility, with the operation itself or with any combination of these.

6.1.3.1 Infection

For the mother recovering from a caesarean, she is vulnerable to infection in one or more of a number of sites. While any infection may carry a threat to the woman's life, maternal deaths due to infection incurred during the surgery are now unusual in developed countries (Harper, 2004:114). The other implications are still serious, though, as the woman may be too unwell to care for herself or to care for and feed her baby. Further, she may need a longer stay in the hospital or admission to the intensive care unit. In the event of a wound infection, it may impede healing, which has additional repercussions in any future pregnancy (please see section 8.3.1).

An audit of the incidence of caesarean wound infections in district general hospitals in the north of England found a rate as low as 6.95 per cent (Nice et al, 1996). The published data demonstrate the association which is ordinarily assumed between postnatal infection and duration of labour, and duration of rupture of membranes and number of vaginal examinations, respectively. These researchers found no significant difference between women who had been administered prophylactic antibiotics and those who had not. Surprisingly, unlike Wrightson (1996), neither was there any significant difference between women having an elective caesarean and those undergoing an emergency operation. These authors conclude that routine prophylaxis is not appropriate and that antibiotics should only be administered prophylactically to women deemed to be at high risk of developing an infection.

While any routine should cause us to pause for thought, routine prophylactic antibiotics in association with a caesarean continues to be a contentious issue. Fears of allergic reactions, of increasing the number of hospital acquired infections and of masking neonatal infection have all been argued against routine prophylaxis (Nice et al, 1996). The contentious nature of this debate is raised in a systematic review of antibiotic prophylaxis (Smaill and Hofmeyr, 2002). This review concludes that all women undergoing caesarean should be recommended to accept prophylactic antibiotics. The authors are at pains to cover all bases, though, by emphasising the importance of observing all of the basic principles of hygiene in order to minimise infection rates. The importance of strict adherence to the principles of hygiene cannot be overemphasised. Perhaps unfortunately, as mentioned in the 2000–02 Confidential Enquiries, a generation of staff is now providing care who have no experience of life-threatening infections (Harper, 2004:116). There is no mention of complacency, but this may become a real possibility, due to over-reliance on routine prophylactic antibiotics with little need to observe the basic principles of infection prevention. Such a self-satisfied attitude was highlighted in the work of Wrightson, who identified the consistent underestimation of the incidence of caesarean wound infections, due simply to a failure to 'send sufficient swabs for examination' (1996:35).

A group of bacteria which have earned themselves the title 'Superbugs', more accurately the methicillin-resistant Staphylococcus aureus (MRSA), have made disconcerting progress into a range of health care facilities. While it is known that maternity facilities are not immune to 'colonisation', childbearing women are less likely than people with long-term health problems to experience MRSA bacteraemia (DoH, 2006). Although a systematic review found no advantage in seeking to eradicate MRSA in colonised individuals, the spread of MRSA 'via colonised hands of healthcare workers' (Loeb et al, 2003) is yet another reminder of the need for continuing vigilance.

6.1.3.2 Thrombo-embolic conditions

Deep vein thrombosis (DVT) and the embolus which may break away from it constitute a major threat to maternal life. A woman's risk of thrombo-embolism is increased six fold by pregnancy and a further 2 to 20 times by caesarean (Jackson and Paterson-Brown, 2001).

A range of physiological mechanisms protect the woman from excessive blood loss during childbirth. These include increased plasma fibrinogen, decreased fibrinolytic activity, increased circulating volume and myometrial contractions (Letsky, 1985). Unfortunately, the first two of these mechanisms may be too effective and put the woman in jeopardy of excessive blood coagulation. Immobility, such as during or after a caesarean, leads to slow circulation in the dependent body parts, such as pelvis or legs, and may be sufficient to initiate clotting or haemostasis.

Thrombosis begins with an aggregation of platelets in a blood vessel, such as the femoral vein, possibly at the site of pre-existing endothelial damage. The thrombus which is formed in this way may not be dangerous as, outwith pregnancy, fibrinolysis would destroy it spontaneously (Hinchliff and Montague, 1988). A surviving thrombus, however, may grow to occlude the lumen of the vessel. The blood beyond this original clot becomes static and coagulates, forming a 'tail' of clot, anchored only at its origin. Clearly, portions of this tail may detach. These are emboli, which may lodge in narrow pulmonary or cerebral arterioles causing dreadful pain, other clinical features and possibly death (Baskett, 1985).

The commonly mentioned complication of DVT is pulmonary embolism (Baskett, 1985; Bonica, 1990). The reason for this focus is unclear in view of the greater risk of cerebral embolism (HMSO, 1996). Pulmonary embolism's bad press is due to the occlusion of the pulmonary circulation by the thrombus, producing hypoxia, acute pulmonary hypertension, right ventricular failure and cardiogenic shock. The local effect of pulmonary occlusion is exacerbated by the production of serotonin, prostaglandins and histamine, which further constrict circulation. While a massive pulmonary embolism may cause the woman to collapse and die, she may survive the initial episode and be transferred for intensive care. Disseminated intravascular coagulation (DIC) may supervene, leading to a 'vicious circle' of clotting and 'disastrous bleeding' (Letsky, 1985:74) in various sites throughout the woman's body.

Although increasing age, a high body mass index, a previous episode and high multiparity have been incriminated as predisposing to thrombo-embolism, caesarean's significant role emerges clearly from the Confidential Enquiries (HMSO, 1996). Of the 17 maternal deaths due to pulmonary embolism within six postnatal weeks, 13 (76 per cent) of the women had given birth by caesarean section.

The main approach to thromboembolic conditions is prevention, using pharmacological prophylaxis (comprising anticoagulant therapy) in women at risk. Additionally, prophylactic therapeutic interventions, such as passive movement and early mobilisation are particularly significant in this group of women. A systematic review, however, found that the existing studies are too small to draw any conclusions about the value of these interventions (Gates et al, 2002). In spite of this, the RCOG Risk Assessment Profile for thrombo-embolism in caesarean section (1995) adopts a flexible approach which may avoid unnecessary medication in many women. This profile seeks to provide individualised prophylaxis depending on the woman's risk status:

1   Low risk: Recommend early mobilisation and hydration. History of:

   • elective caesarean
   • uncomplicated pregnancy and no other risk factors.

2   Moderate risk: Consider one of a variety of prophylactic measures such as subcutaneous heparin or mechanical methods. History of:

   • age >35 years
   • obesity (>80 kg)
   • parity 4 or more
   • labour 12 hours or more
   • gross varicose veins
   • current infection
   • pre-eclampsia
   • immobility prior to surgery (>4 days)
   • major current illness (e.g. heart or lung disease, cancer, inflammatory bowel disease, nephrotic syndrome)
   • emergency caesarean in labour.

3   High risk: Recommend heparin prophylaxis with or without leg stockings. Prophylaxis until the fifth postoperative day is advised (or until fully mobilised if longer). History of:

- three or more moderate risk factors from above
- extended major pelvic or abdominal surgery (e.g. caesarean hysterectomy)
- personal or family history of deep venous thrombosis, pulmonary embolism or thrombophilia, paralysis of lower limbs
- antiphospholipid antibody (cardiolipin antibody or lupus anticoagulant).

It is an unfortunate reflection on the state of obstetric research that the most common cause of direct maternal deaths, thrombo-embolism, does not yet have a sound evidence base on which practice may be founded (Lewis, 2004:26).

6.1.3.3 Bowel function

Although Jackson and Paterson-Brown describe damage to the bowel during caesarean as 'very rare' (2001:55), the Confidential Enquiries for 2000–02 included five deaths due to perforation of the bowel. All of these deaths followed caesareans, but for four of these women, there was no damage to the bowel at time of operation. In three of the women, a diagnosis of Ogilvie's syndrome was made, which is an 'acute pseudo-obstruction' of the colon (Smith, 2006). In this condition, there is no mechanical obstruction, but the peristalsis of the bowel is either reduced or absent. For this reason, the differential diagnosis is '*adynamic* or *paralytic ileus*'. Ogilvie's syndrome mimics intestinal obstruction in that the bowel becomes distended with gases and fluid; because of the severity of the distension, it may eventually perforate, which was the cause of death in three of the women (Drife, 2004:120).

The cause of these conditions is uncertain, but there has been a traditional assumption that the onset is linked to early eating and drinking postoperatively. For this reason, food and fluids have often been withheld (see section 6.1.2.3). A controlled trial suggests that withholding oral intake is not justified (Gocmen et al, 2002). In the sample of 182 women undergoing caesarean, the incidence of paralytic ileus was 5.3 per cent (n=5) in the early fed group and 6.9 (n=6) in the traditionally fed group. Other suggested causes of paralytic ileus include manipulation of the bowel and suturing of the peritoneum during the caesarean (Jackson and Paterson-Brown, 2001:55).

Ogilvie's syndrome is more commonly associated with caesarean than with any other form of surgery and is more likely to be fatal than paralytic ileus (Roberts et al, 2000). That Ogilvie's syndrome may be caused by sympathetic/parasympathetic imbalance has long been assumed (Ogilvie, 1948:672). The link with certain forms of pain control, such as epidural and general anaesthetic, is a more recent belief (Roberts et al, 2000). The increasing incidence of Ogilvie's syndrome demonstrates, once again, how the spectre of iatrogenesis may manifest itself.

In his report, Drife draws attention to the problem of diagnosing intestinal obstruction in the early days after caesarean. When the diagnosis was made in three of the cases, the relatively junior medical staff failed to recognise the serious nature of this condition in a new mother. In another woman's case, she had been transferred home and the community midwives did not record any abdominal distension. Drife correctly observes that many midwives are not general nurses; but he then proceeds to recommend that 'attention must be paid to education of midwives in postoperative management' (2004:121). This example of scapegoating is unwarranted from such a heavily medically dominated panel of assessors. Perhaps the 'follow up' referred to by NICE (see section 6.1.2.2) seeks to allocate a responsibility to community midwifery which this service is neither prepared nor staffed to assume.

6.1.4 The emotional response

In this chapter, the focus is on the implications for the woman and the baby in the period during and immediately after the caesarean. The time period has, so far, not needed to be defined because the issues addressed have had a relatively short and fixed time span. These implications arise within, at most, two weeks of the birth and probably while the midwife continues to visit. In considering the woman's emotional response, though, the picture is somewhat different. This point is addressed in a discussion of the woman's 'early emotional recovery' from caesarean (Clement, 1995). She draws an analogy between the healing of the caesarean wound and the 'wound in our mind' (1995:83); she maintains that the healing of the former is by far the speedier. The woman's slow emotional recovery is, according to Clement, due to her state of shock in the early days; this is a state which probably lasts for the duration of her stay in the maternity unit. Her emotional shock allows the woman to do little more on an emotional level than repeat the mantra which is being fed to her of how lucky she is to have such a beautiful baby.

This point is reinforced by Oakley in the context of a survey accessing women's views of their pain control in labour (1993). She showed that collecting data during the woman's stay in the maternity unit is of little value. She estimated that the time taken for the woman to come to terms with her feelings sufficiently to answer questions would be about six weeks. This is the reason why Oakley's follow-up survey was infinitely more informative than the data collected earlier.

Because of this initial psychological shock, I address the woman's emotional responses in detail in the chapter on the long-term implications (see section 7.1.2).

6.2 The implications for the baby

As I have already mentioned in Chapter 5 (section 5.5), the welfare of the baby may be the most significant factor in the decision to undertake a caesarean. It may be assumed, therefore, that caesarean can be of nothing but benefit to the baby. In this section, I seek to assess whether and to what extent this assumption of benefit to the baby actually applies.

6.2.1 *Respiratory distress syndrome*

There is a certain attraction in the simple logic of a baby whose thorax is squeezed through the pelvis being less likely to develop respiratory distress. So, it may come as a surprise that, for whatever reason, the benefits of vaginal birth to neonatal pulmonary function are well established. A North American study showed that risks of transient tachypnoea and respiratory distress were greater, even among babies born by elective caesarean (Hook et al, 1997). The comparison group comprised babies born vaginally following a trial of labour. The risks of neonatal respiratory problems were found to correlate negatively with increasing gestational age.

On the basis of these US findings, researchers in Scotland audited a guideline to delay elective caesarean until at least 39 weeks' gestation (Nicoll et al, 2003). This audit demonstrated an impressive reduction in neonatal morbidity. The issue which is particularly interesting, however, is that in spite of general agreement to this guideline, more than one quarter (26 per cent) of elective caesareans continued to be performed before 39 weeks. This observation casts serious doubt on the assumption, noted above, of the benefits of caesarean to the baby. Clearly early elective caesareans are continuing to be performed in spite of the known established risks to the baby. It should be noted, though, that even after the 39-week watershed, the risks of neonatal respiratory morbidity still persist.

6.2.2 *Attachment and separation*

The ground-breaking, although methodologically flawed, work of Klaus and Kennell (1982) demonstrated the significance of early bonding and attachment in human relationships, and its place in maternity care. The risk of interfering with these processes through separation is markedly increased if a caesarean is performed (Buckley, 2004). This separation may be physical, such as when the baby is admitted to the neonatal unit for observation or if the baby is, albeit briefly, transferred to the baby resuscitation room for a paediatric check. Alternatively, the separation may be pharmacological, when the woman and/or the baby are 'out of it' due to opioid analgesics or general anaesthesia. Buckley emphasises the endocrinological implications for both woman and baby of early separation. These implications are closely related to the time when the baby is first put to the breast. For babies born vaginally this crucially important initial interaction happens, on average, one hour and fifteen minutes after the birth. For the baby born by caesarean, though, the average time when that first breast feed happens is four hours after the birth. Thus, for the caesarean baby, that crucial period immediately after the birth, when the baby is supremely sensitive and responsive, is more likely to be spent apart from her mother.

6.2.3 Breast feeding

I have already referred briefly to the challenges facing the mother in caring for her baby after a caesarean (please see section 6.1.2.4). These challenges apply no less to the woman breast feeding her baby after a caesarean. The benefits of breast feeding to the baby are indisputable (Wilson et al, 1998). This is but one reason for encouraging the mother to breast feed and for beginning the initiation of breast feeding as early as possible. A particularly large proportion of women who have caesareans have been shown to be keen to breast feed (Churchill et al, 2006). This should come as no surprise in view of the well-recognised tendencies for more affluent women to both have caesareans and to breast feed (Alves and Sheikh, 2005). As mentioned already, extra pairs of hands are much needed by a new mother embarking on breast feeding, but the crucial physical and psychological state of mind may be even more hard to find. It may be a reflection of the enthusiasm of neonatal staff, that women with babies in the neonatal unit are no more likely to give up breast feeding in the first days and weeks than others (Churchill et al, 2006). These researchers asked the women in their sample whether having had a caesarean was felt to have affected their ability to breast feed. That one fifth of the women replied 'Yes' to this question and that the effect was invariably adverse is a sad evaluation of our maternity services.

6.2.4 Iatrogenic prematurity

Although some may wonder whether the woman might actually be relieved to have her pregnancy foreshortened by an intervention like caesarean, the risks for the baby should never be overlooked. Methods of gestational assessment, such as ultrasound scans, are widely thought to be infallible (Wagner, 2000). The possibility of an elective caesarean erroneously being performed prematurely and delivering a pre-term baby, however, has not been completely overcome (Miller et al, 1996; Maynard et al, 2005). Prematurity brings with it a range of problems, especially for the baby. The problems include respiratory and feeding difficulties, jaundice, gastro-intestinal pathology, separation and prolonged hospitalisation. These outcomes may be further examples of the baby, rather than the obstetrician, being put at risk when a caesarean is performed (Wagner, 2000). Of course, these neonatal problems do not just affect the baby, as the family implications should not be overlooked.

6.2.5 Accidental fetal laceration

The possibility of the surgeon causing laceration to the fetus has become increasingly significant since it was first described by Gerber in 1974. This significance is partly due to the rising caesarean rate and partly to the legal costs which are likely to follow such an accident (Herbert, 2003). The risk of this form of injury is difficult to assess, but the figure is ordinarily quoted at about 0.7 to 1.9 per cent. This is likely to be an underestimate due to under-recording because there is no clear responsibility for logging such injuries (Smith et al, 1997). In the case of the obstetrician, this omission is because the obstetrician may be unaware that the injury has occurred (Herbert, 2003). Interestingly, Herbert argues that as soon as the baby is born the focus of the obstetrician's interest is transferred solely to the mother. In spite of this, Smith and colleagues found that, for some unknown reason, the paediatricians, who were present for all caesareans, recorded only 70 per cent (n=10) of the number of lacerations that the nursing staff recorded (n=17).

Dessole and colleagues' study attempted to correct this tendency to underestimate the frequency of lacerations (2004). Although these researchers claim to have been stringent, their data still relied on the staff present at the birth. Thus, this group's disconcertingly high finding of a fetal laceration rate of 3.12 per cent may also be an underestimate. More helpfully, Dessole and colleagues clearly demonstrate the severity of the lacerations sustained. Unsurprisingly, a large majority of the 97 lacerations (n=94) were categorised as 'mild' (2004:1675). These mild lacerations, though, were sufficient to need to have a 'sterile strip' (2004:1675) applied. Additionally 21 of the mild lacerations affected the face or ear. Though recorded as 'mild' lacerations, scarring was still visible at a six-month follow up. The Dessole et al series included two cases of 'moderate' lacerations, measuring 2 cm and 4 cm in length. The shorter affected the face and the longer the baby's neck. In both of these babies, cosmetic surgery was required but scarring persisted. The one baby who sustained a severe laceration was presenting as a breech; the laceration measured 5 cm long and involved superficial, muscle and nervous tissues.

Perhaps in an attempt to reduce the impact of their findings, Dessole and colleagues argue that such injuries may be a small price to pay to 'avoid the risk of fetal morbidity and death' (2004:1676). In a similarly cavalier fashion, the seriousness of this problem further appears to be dismissed when it is reported that there were no 'functional sequelae' (2004:1676). An element of defensiveness creeps in when the recommendation is made that the possibility of fetal laceration should be mentioned to the woman when she gives consent for the caesarean (Dessole et al, 2004:1673; Herbert, 2003:9).

One aspect of fetal laceration, which I have not yet located in the literature, is its significance when the caesarean is being performed to avoid vertical transmission of a blood-borne infection. Clearly, a fetal laceration would compromise the baby's protection from infection, defeating the entire purpose of the surgery.

Thus, it would appear that the mother may not be the only person to leave the operating theatre with a wound to show for the time spent there.

6.3 Mother and baby

Unlike the woman who gives birth vaginally, the one who has a caesarean can only give birth in hospital. Additionally, while recognising that the hospital stay for all women and their babies is becoming shorter, for the woman who gives birth by caesarean this stay is inevitably longer. Petrou and colleagues (2001) found that in one English health region the hospital stay following a caesarean was three times the length of stay after a spontaneous birth. Some of the joys and risks of hospitalisation have been explored already (see section 6.1.2.2). It is necessary to bear in mind, though, that while some women may appreciate the support and security offered by the staff in a maternity unit, others may see it differently. For some women the longer hospital stay may be socially inconvenient or even unpleasant. This may be due to separation from home and family or to the difficulty of beginning to establish routines in an alien hospital environment. For still others, this time spent in the maternity unit may not be without risk.

One of these risks is the group of infections, formerly termed 'nosocomial', which have become known as the HAIs or Hospital Acquired/Health Associated Infections (see section 3.3.1.4). The risks of infection to a woman who is recovering from a caesarean are many, including respiratory, uterine and urinary infections (Thomas, 2000). The risks to her baby attract little attention (Jackson and Paterson-Brown, 2001), but include additional gastro-intestinal and skin infections. Many of the endeavours to reduce the incidence of HAIs has focused, first, on visitors and, second, on nursing staff (SE, 2006). The effectiveness of such approaches remains to be seen. It would appear to be little more than common sense, though, that a woman and baby who are either not admitted or are hospitalised for a shorter period of time are at reduced risk of contracting hospital acquired infections.

6.4 Maternal mortality

In this chapter up to this point, I have considered some of the problems which the woman and her baby may encounter during or immediately after a caesarean operation. It is now necessary to consider the meaning of these outcomes. One of these is maternal death, the spectre of which has manifested itself already in relation to a number of aspects of the woman's experience (please see section 5.3.3). My own research has shown that this topic constitutes a deeply feared taboo among midwives (Mander, 2001b). It may be that this fearful taboo is related to the widely held perception of maternity and midwifery being happy areas in which to practise. Midwives and others have gone to great lengths to persuade childbearing families of the healthy and normal nature of childbearing. Obviously, the death of a mother is the absolute antithesis of such perceptions. It may be that midwives have been so successful in persuading others of the healthy nature of childbearing that it has become unacceptable for the midwife to even contemplate the possibility of a mother dying. Bearing this in mind, it is difficult to imagine that childbearing women appreciate the extent to which caesarean increases the risk of maternal death. The extent of this increase has been estimated variously to be between two-fold and eleven-fold (Hillan, 2000).

The significance of maternal mortality varies according to the local environment or culture. It invariably involves the death of a woman who has been, at least, young and healthy enough to become pregnant. In some less developed countries, where the problem is numerically greater, maternal death may be associated with the status of women in society, with their education and with the balance of power between men and women. In developed countries, where the maternal mortality rate is generally lower, these issues may be less significant. There are, however, other issues which assume considerably greater importance, even when the maternal mortality statistics are numerically low. These issues relate to the appropriateness of treatments or interventions to which women are subjected or allow themselves to be subjected. In the event of treatment which may be inappropriate, harm may ensue. Because of this possibility, it is now necessary to focus on the concept incorporating such harm.

6.5 Iatrogenesis

Although the word itself is not yet in popular usage, the phenomenon which is iatrogenesis has been increasingly recognised in health care since ancient times (Penn, 1986). For the introduction of the word itself, we are indebted to Illich (1976). He explains that it is derived from the Greek words *iatros*, meaning physician, and *genesis*, meaning origin (1976:11). This word emerged out of his analysis of a number of institutions, including medicine and education, which proved to be counter-productive in terms of their intended goals (Illich, 1995). Thus, Illich applied this concept solely to medical personnel, rather than the now wider application to professional health care staff. The importance of iatrogenesis was underscored a short while later by the introduction of its antonym *salutogenesis*, by Antonovsky in 1979.

Historically, iatrogenesis is a concept which has traditionally been applied to pharmacology, which is Penn's main focus (1986); it applies no less to maternity, though. This applicability is demonstrated in a short yet dishonourable list of the drugs, devices and interventions causing iatrogenic conditions, including thalidomide, the Dalkon Shield, routine episiotomy and diethylstiboestrol (DES).

Although usually literally translated as 'illness induced by the physician' (Sharpe and Faden, 1998:1), in a clinical setting iatrogenesis means harm in the course of treatment. It may be argued that in certain circumstances caesarean may actually be an iatrogenic intervention. Some of the short-term implications for the woman, which feature life-threatening complications, have been mentioned already in this chapter. They include adverse events during and after surgery, such as haemorrhage, thrombo-embolic conditions and infection. Also during surgery, problems relating to awareness or the partner not being permitted to be present for the birth, do not affect the woman's physical health *per se*, but are certainly likely to harm the quality of her childbirth experience.

In this section, I probe whether and to what extent the term iatrogenesis is applicable to caesarean. In his profoundly disturbing analysis of the consequences of professional health care interventions, Illich identified three major areas of concern. First, he focused on what he termed 'clinical iatrogenesis' (1976:21), by which he meant harm caused directly by supposedly therapeutic interventions. By way of an example of how medicine achieved its high status, he cites the well-known demise of the tubercle bacillus (TB) in the 1930s. While this success has been claimed as a medical breakthrough, Illich demonstrates that the sulphonamides were little more than the *coup de grâce* to a seriously incapacitated organism.

After exposing such unfounded claims to the benefits of science, he goes on to examine useless interventions and then 'doctor-inflicted injuries'. In the latter category, he cites the development of infections, some of which are drug resistant, and the medical diagnosis of 'non-diseases'. These are highly pertinent in the caesarean debate. As mentioned already, infection is a cause of post-caesarean morbidity in both the woman and her baby (see section 6.1.3.1). For this reason the title 'doctor-inflicted injury' may be apposite. Similarly, as shown in Chapter 5, many of the so-called 'indications' for caesarean have no basis in research evidence and may, therefore, be classified as 'non-diseases'. Examples would include failure to progress/dystocia, breech presentation and many cases diagnosed as fetal distress. Thus, because of the wide range of risks inherent in caesarean mentioned already, the woman's health, and possibly her life, may be being put in jeopardy for some reason other than her or her baby's welfare.

The second focus of Illich's scrutiny is 'social iatrogenesis'. By this he is referring to the various forms of harm that result from the 'socio-economic transformations which have been made attractive, possible or necessary' by health services developing professional and institutional structures and systems (1976:49). Particularly insidious is the way in which medicine has removed from communities the ability to care for their own, by effectively de-skilling the people who have traditionally provided support and emergency aid. In this way, health services have created a dependent group of patients or clients. Among the members of this group, the expectations and demands are infinite, yet they have minimal power to evaluate the effectiveness of any care provided. The relevance of social iatrogenesis to caesarean is clearly apparent. This phenomenon is found in the acceptance of and demand for the caesarean operation, particularly in situations where the rationale is flimsy, to the point of being non-existent.

The third aspect of iatrogenesis which is explored by Illich is 'cultural iatrogenesis'. Rather than the effects on individuals, this phenomenon affects the attitudes of an entire cultural group, perhaps even a complete generation. The attitudes involved are those involving the fundamental aspects of human existence, such as infirmity and frail old age. These are the aspects which medicine seeks to prevent at all costs. Significant in the present context are the changing attitudes to suffering and pain, which are regarded as the ultimate adversaries, to be strenuously avoided. Of course, with medical intervention suffering and pain, such as those inherent in labour, can supposedly be eradicated. In this way, cultural iatrogenesis serves to increase the likelihood of caesarean by limiting the woman's preparedness to face the challenges of labouring and giving birth spontaneously.

One of the crucial strategies in bringing about cultural iatrogenesis is the manipulation of language:

> Language is taken over by the doctors: the sick person is deprived of meaningful words for his [*sic*] anguish, which is thus further increased by linguistic mystification.

> (Illich 1976:175)

The manipulation of language happens at a number of different levels. Initially, the consumer of health care is made to doubt the healthy functioning of her own body. This is through negative messages which have become standard through the widespread mimicry of medical jargon. Such terminology includes, for example:

> failure to progress
> incompetent cervix
> habitual abortion
> elderly primigravida

These examples of medical jargon serve to aggravate any doubts which the woman may be harbouring about her own ability to give birth healthily and spontaneously. The next stage of manipulation of language involves the normalisation of certain quite extreme interventions in order to overcome the perceived failure. In this way, the woman is lulled into believing that, in the likely event of her inability to give birth as she wishes, the 'rescue operation' is little more than routine and humdrum. Hence, the previously technical jargon, such as 'c-section', 'caesar' or 'section', become little more than colloquialisms. In this way the threshold to performing the caesarean is lowered even further.

For obvious reasons, Illich and his ideas have been vilified, largely on the grounds that his case is seriously overstated. I would venture to suggest, though, that there is more than a little resonance between Illich's three forms of iatrogenesis and the changing practices of and views about caesarean.

A North American analysis of forms of surgery which may be categorised as iatrogenic includes some caesareans (Sharpe and Faden, 1998). These authors describe the 'general skepticism' (1998:194) that surgery which is unnecessary ever actually happens. The reverse assumption all too often prevails – that if surgery has been performed, then it must have been necessary. The argument is then moved forward to demonstrate the inevitably iatrogenic nature of unnecessary surgery. Sharpe and Faden admit that unnecessary surgery exposes the patient to unjustified and unjustifiable risks, quoting specifically hospital acquired infection and adverse anaesthesia-related events. They argue, though, that even in the absence of such pathological outcomes the very fact of an invasive intervention, such as surgery, being performed unnecessarily is '*de facto* harmful' (1998:194, italics in original).

After establishing the damaging nature of unnecessary surgery and the fact that it occurs, Sharpe and Faden go on to search for the reasons why it still continues. The answer is found in the supply and demand issues, which manifest themselves in the 'medical marketplace' (1998:205). These issues are particularly relevant in the context of caesarean because of the link with the fashionable or 'fad operations' (1998:205). These authors cite other forms of fashionable surgery which have, like caesarean, become particularly popular among the wealthier sections of the community (see Chapter 4); their longstanding examples include childhood tonsillectomy. Because of their North American origins Sharpe and Faden dwell at length on the financial incentives to perform unnecessary surgery. I would suggest that, at the time of writing, financial remuneration is still not a major factor in the

UK. It is necessary to question, though, whether the high social status of being an obstetric *surgeon* serves as some kind of proxy. These authors' other reasons for the persistence of unnecessary surgery have been addressed elsewhere, and include defensive medicine and an inadequate evidence or knowledge base.

In the next chapter (Chapter 7), I address the longer-term outcomes associated with caesarean, which further reinforce the iatrogenic nature of this form of intervention.

6.6 Conclusion

In this chapter, I have demonstrated some of the problems which the woman may encounter during and immediately after a birth by caesarean. These problems have ranged broadly in terms of their effects on the mother and the baby's health and well-being. They have also varied in the likelihood of their occurrence. Of necessity, I have had to mention the possibility of these problems being associated with the death of the woman.

The message which emerges out of this examination of these problems is that caesarean is by no means a risk-free mode of birth. The nature of these risks is such that it may be concluded that they are associated with the operation itself. For this reason, the possibility of caesarean being a form of iatrogenesis has been considered. The conclusion which emerges is that caesarean may be seen to accord with the three types of iatrogenesis proposed by Illich (1976).

7   The long-term implications of caesarean

Through the medium of this book, I am seeking to explore the reputation which caesarean has for being a 'quick fix' and the extent to which this reputation is deserved. As well as the immediate implications which were discussed in Chapter 6, there may be others of a longer duration. Thus, this surgical operation may yet prove to be neither a fix nor quick. This contention is supported by women who have previously had a caesarean and often find themselves surprised to find how quickly they recover from a spontaneous birth. The validity of such comparisons is not certain, because the woman may not be comparing like with like. The point is well made, though, that recovery from a caesarean operation is all too different from recovery after a physiological birth.

In contemplating the long-term implications, it is crucial to keep in mind the woman's situation. By this, I mean that in physical terms the woman is recovering from major abdominal surgery. For this reason, both her internal and her superficial wounds need to be allowed to complete their healing processes. In addition, she has a new baby or babies, who require attention day and night. She also has all the usual womanly tasks which she may not have been able or prepared to off-load on to those close to her. As well as the physical wounds and challenges, this woman faces all of the emotional and relational adjustments which a new family member brings; these are on top of any lingering uncertainty about her mode of giving birth. It is apparent that the caesarean-related implications are superimposed on what can only be described as this woman's busy schedule.

In this chapter, against this background of recovery, adjustment and change, I examine some of the problems which have been shown by research to be associated with a surgical birth. As has been the predominant focus of this book, the woman's experience is the major concern. Inevitably, though, others are affected on a long-term basis by the increasing incidence of caesarean. The effects for the baby come easily to mind. Additionally, there are the implications for health care providers and also for the groups which are becoming and have become established for the woman who has experienced a caesarean.

As we consider this woman's birth experience and her recovery from it, it is essential to keep sight of the individual nature of any birth. If two women have an apparently similar birth experience, there is no reason why they should both share the same feelings about and reactions to it. Each woman will bring her own hopes, expectations and aspirations, as well as all of her own emotional baggage. These factors will inevitably colour her perception of her experience. In this way, each woman may be more satisfied or more disappointed with the events surrounding the birth of her baby.

7.1 Implications for the woman

As mentioned in the introduction to this chapter, following a caesarean the woman faces a multitude of challenges. The development of caesarean-related health problems can only aggravate the difficulties that face her. In this section, I consider some of these problems. Initially, though, it is necessary to contemplate the significance of these problems to the woman. Each health problem brings with it its own specific impact, but generally such problems add yet another burden to those facing her. An example would be, as found in a study in Australia (Thompson et al, 2002), the significantly greater difficulty which caesarean mothers encounter in coping with their exhaustion or extreme tiredness. The woman's difficulties really escalate, though, if the health problem is such that readmission to hospital becomes necessary. As mentioned already (see section 6.3), the hospital environment is not without risks, which include psychosocial problems as well as the physical ones.

The size of the problem of readmission postnatally emerged in a large and authoritative research project which was undertaken in Washington State, USA (Lydon-Rochelle et al, 2000). To study first time mothers who were readmitted following the birth, quantitative data were collected from 971 women seven weeks after giving birth. These researchers found the usual positive correlation between social class and giving birth by caesarean. Of particular significance was the finding that following a caesarean, the woman was almost twice as likely to be readmitted, compared with the woman who had a spontaneous birth. In an Australian study, however, the proportion of readmissions was 5.3 per cent of caesarean mothers compared with 2.2 per cent in other groups. In the survey in Washington State, wound complications was by far the most common reason for readmission. Caesarean wounds were 30 times more likely to be the indication for readmission than the other wounds which the woman may sustain during, for example, a spontaneous birth. Although a long way behind, infectious and thrombo-embolic conditions were the next most common indications for readmission. On the basis of these findings the American researchers make a plea for more appropriate use of obstetric interventions.

It may be that hospital readmission is regarded as an extreme example of the problems which a woman faces post caesarean. Other publications by this team of American researchers, though, show that the occurrence of this event is not markedly different from the general picture of this woman's health (Lydon-Rochelle et al, 2001). The woman who had had a caesarean was found to score significantly lower on a range of aspects of physical functioning than her peer who had given birth spontaneously.

7.1.1 Post-caesarean pain

In the work of the Washington State group (Lydon-Rochelle et al, 2001) the major factor which impeded the caesarean mother's physical functioning was her continuing bodily pain. The extent to which the woman's pain is able to be controlled in the early post-caesarean period has been addressed already (see section 6.1.2.1). That the early difficulties continue for some women in the form of incapacitating pain has long been clearly established (Hillan, 1992b). In her ground-breaking project, this researcher applied a postal questionnaire at twelve weeks after the birth to a large cohort of women who had given birth by caesarean (n=444). Hillan found that, for almost half of the women, their wound pain lasted well beyond their transfer home, which was then at least five days after the operation. The severity of the wound pain after leaving hospital was sufficient to require the administration of 'prescription only' analgesic medication in 11.7 per cent of the women (n=52). Of these women, 32 were still experiencing wound pain when they completed the questionnaire at twelve weeks. These longer-term data reinforce the findings on the woman's experience of immediate postoperative pain, in that both groups' pain problems were denigrated by the health care staff. Hillan (1992b) was able to compare the women's reports of their experience with midwifery and medical records. Although 43 per cent of the women reported back pain and 12 per cent reported painful haemorrhoids, these problems were recorded in only 8 per cent and none, respectively, of the women's notes. These data lead to the conclusion that for the midwifery staff, as found by Willson among a sample of nurses (2000), there were other agendas operating.

There may be a temptation to disregard the findings of Hillan's late twentieth-century study on the grounds of their age. These findings are, however, endorsed by more recent work in Denmark, which was undertaken because of the absence of research on chronic pain after 'gynaecologic surgery' (Nikolajsen et al, 2004: 111). These researchers undertook a survey of all women who had given birth by caesarean in one Danish maternity unit in a twelve-month period (n=245). One of the women had died. The postal questionnaire asked for demographic information as well as details of any ongoing caesarean-related pain. The importance of these issues to women is apparent in the response rate to the questionnaire. The women, who were obviously extremely busy because they had given birth 6 to 17.2 months earlier, were so concerned about post-caesarean pain control that the response rate reached the amazingly high figure of 90.2 per cent (n=220).

These Danish researchers found that for a small majority of women (55 per cent, n=121) the postoperative pain had lasted for not more than one month. Almost one quarter of the women experienced postoperative pain lasting between one and three months. For 12.3 per cent of the women (n=27), however, the pain was still present when they responded to the questionnaire. Thus, these recent findings more than support what Hillan found in 1992. The Danish researchers, being anaesthetists, gave little attention to the impact of their pain on the women's lives. They did elicit, though, that it had a (presumably adverse) influence on a range of daily activities. These routine activities which were hampered included carrying something heavy;

because a young baby fits that description, the woman's activities would be seriously curtailed. Unsurprisingly, the Danish study also found that the pain affected the woman's mood and that she had to resort to pain medication.

Nikolajsen and colleagues were able to identify some factors which they thought might be associated with continuing pain. One of these is the caesarean having been performed under general anaesthesia. They attribute this link to the possibility of a 'traumatic memory' (2004:114) of an emergency caesarean. Further, the women with continuing pain were significantly more likely to be experiencing pain in other parts of their bodies. The researchers go as far as to attribute this finding to 'psychosocial factors' or to 'preoperative neuroticism' (2004:114). It would appear that, although these researchers examined this phenomenon admirably carefully, their analysis of the causes is, to say the least, cavalier.

The significance of post-caesarean pain is taken more seriously in the work of Churchill (2003). She contrasts the woman's expectations with the reality, because she does not expect to become an 'invalid' or to be 'immobilised by major surgery' (2003:142). Nor does the woman's self-esteem survive unscathed: 'I couldn't quite manage because of the pain I was in. It left me feeling inadequate as a mother, and I wanted to do more' (2003:142).

Thus, it is clear that neither the severity nor the duration of post-caesarean pain are being given the research attention and the clinical attention which is obviously justified. The 'other agendas', which Willson (2000) identified during the hospital stay, may also apply to the woman's experience of longer-term pain.

The possibility of long-term post-caesarean wound pain being due to a less obvious cause has been raised by Olufowobi and colleagues (2003). These authors report the case of a woman who experienced a painful swelling adjacent to her caesarean scar; the severity of the pain became worse during her menstrual periods. After three years, the scar was investigated and the swelling was found to contain endometrial tissue. These cells had been transferred from the uterus during the caesarean and were responding to her monthly cycle, just as the uterine lining does. After removal of the swelling, the woman's pain was resolved. The writers observe that, in association with the rising caesarean rate, it may be necessary for health care personnel to consider the possibility of endometriosis if and when a woman complains of long-term post-caesarean wound pain.

7.1.2 Emotional implications

The escalation in the caesarean rate has occurred concurrently with marked changes in women's attitudes to birth. The recent rise in women's expectations has been linked to the information now widely available regarding the choices which the woman may face (Hillan, 2000). These expectations can only have been fuelled by statements from a range of agencies, including governmental bodies (DoH, 1993). Obviously, the reaction of the individual woman to her caesarean will vary according to a wide range of factors. These include her attitudes, expectations and aspirations, not to mention her actual birth experience. Any variations will apply to the time frame as well as to the nature and the occurrence of any emotional reactions.

The inability of childbearing women to engage with their carers has been shown to result in expectations and aspirations being dashed (Green and Baston, 2003; McCourt and Pearce, 2000:151). Thus, if a woman's expectations of healthy, satisfying childbearing deteriorate into a complicated and/or traumatic and/or surgical birth, they are different again. The role of the woman's culture in the building up of her expectations is crucial. Hence, the importance of culturally sensitive care in the achievement of a satisfying birth experience should never be underestimated (Adewuya et al, 2006).

If the woman's expectations fail to be fulfilled by her experience, this constitutes a form of loss. In this event a number of emotional reactions may be expected to emerge, of which post traumatic stress disorder (PTSD) is but one. Early work in this area was brought together by a ground-breaking research project by Menage (1993). Although this research involved the use of a volunteer sample, Menage was able to identify the obstetric and gynaecological procedures which are likely to be sufficiently traumatic to engender PTSD. The procedures themselves may appear relatively trivial to a professional health care provider, including taking a cervical smear, induction of labour and removing an intrauterine contraceptive device (IUCD). Perhaps more importantly, Menage identified the factors which aggravated the perception of trauma, such as the attendant being male and the existence of a sexual component. This research found that the woman's perception of control of the situation is fundamentally important. Her control may be as basic as knowing that the attendant will stop what they are doing if and when asked.

Menage concluded that she was unable to ascertain whether the trauma of the intervention was totally due to the intervention itself, or whether the woman had been sensitised during a previous experience. This dilemma was addressed in a questionnaire survey of 289 women in London (Ayers and Pickering, 2001). The existence and level of PTSD was ascertained and measured at 36 weeks' gestation and at 6 weeks and 6 months postnatally. During pregnancy 6.2 per cent of the women (n=18) were found to have PTSD and were excluded from subsequent data analysis. Seven new cases of PTSD were identified at six weeks, suggesting that the experience of birth is actually a trigger factor for PTSD. These quantitative studies have been criticised because the instruments had been designed for use following war and other large-scale conflicts in which men were predominantly involved (Moyzakitis, 2004). This critique went on to identify the vulnerable women and the interventions in childbearing which could result in the new mother feeling traumatised. Such trauma may be doubly significant, because it not only affects the woman's emotional state, but also jeopardises fledgling family relationships (Beech, 1998/99).

Although the significance of the trauma to the new mother appears clear, research into her care is less so. 'Debriefing' has been widely welcomed as the solution to any number of postnatal problems (Steele and Beadle, 2003); its precise nature and aims, though, remain unclear. The role of the midwife has been demonstrated in reducing postnatal depression (Lavender and Walkinshaw, 1998; Small et al, 2000), but these interventions do not yet appear to have been applied to new mothers with PTSD (Joseph and Bailham, 2004).

In an examination of the emotional repercussions of caesarean, it emerges that a grief reaction may be appropriate (Lowdon, 1995a). While the mother grieving the loss of her hoped for experience of uncomplicated childbearing (Mander, 2006b) may be regarded as 'selfish', Lowdon considers that it is a coping strategy. She argues, though, that such coping is a fragile strategy which may be threatened by any possibility that the caesarean may not have been 'absolutely necessary' (1995a:14). Further, Lowdon details the anxiety of the mother who is uncertain about whether she has actually been given her own baby. While such anxieties may have been standard, and possibly justified, when general anaesthesia was routinely used for caesarean, it is not certain that this still applies. On the basis of these emotional after shocks, Lowdon rightly pleads that space and time should be made for the woman to articulate not only the gratitude which is usually forthcoming, but also her doubts and confusion.

This picture of not just less satisfaction, but more confusion and traumatisation following a caesarean is generally supported by the research literature (Clement, 2001). Comparison with women having a vaginal birth (DiMatteo et al, 1996) suggests that the difference is significant. The situation regarding postnatal depression after caesarean, though, is somewhat less straightforward. While many studies indicate that the woman is more likely to become depressed after a caesarean than after a vaginal birth, there are almost as many studies which suggest no real difference (Clement, 2001). The conclusion is that the type of birth may have some effect, but that that effect is small. There are other factors which have been shown more clearly to exert more marked effects, including poor psychosocial support, personal psychiatric history and a generally stressful life.

Although the effect of caesarean itself is not entirely clear, emergency as opposed to elective caesarean has been shown to carry a poorer psychological prognosis. The lack of preparation time for the emergency operation has been blamed for these adverse psychological outcomes (Clement, 2001). Similarly, and possibly for the same reasons, psychological problems have been shown to be less likely if the caesarean is undertaken using a regional anaesthetic rather than general anaesthesia. Research in Sweden was crucial in demonstrating the extent of the psychological trauma associated with an emergency caesarean under general anaesthesia (Ryding et al, 1998). This study examined the emotional responses of 53 new mothers, using quantitative techniques. The emotional trauma of an emergency caesarean under general anaesthesia was found to be sufficient to fulfil the stressor criteria for PTSD. The women articulated having experienced feelings of guilt, anger, ignorance and having been abused.

The risk of postnatal depression following emergency caesarean has led some to conclude that, for the woman who may be particularly vulnerable, a prophylactic caesarean may be appropriate. In an effort to study whether elective caesarean was protective against depression, Patel and colleagues (2005) undertook a prospective population-based cohort study involving 14,663 women. The rationale for this study was linked primarily to the intellectual and behavioural development of the baby/child. These researchers found that caesarean offers no protection against postnatal depression, so there is no reason to plan the care of the vulnerable woman differently from the care of others.

As well as the possibility of either PTSD or postnatal depression, which are measurable quantitatively, there remain the less tangible forms of distress which may follow caesarean. These emerge out of the questionnaire-based study by Clement (1995; 2001) which collected the feelings and impressions of 200 women. The informants were recruited through a parents' magazine and childbirth education organisations.

Some of the women who responded to Clement's questionnaire reported 'overwhelming' *loss* (Clement, 2001:117). The focus of the woman's loss related to (i) not experiencing the birth for which they had planned and hoped or (ii) not being able to give birth actively herself or (iii) not actually 'being there' if general anaesthesia was used for the caesarean. Thus, the loss of the birthing experience may be a source of profound regret. The loss of the experience is closely linked to the fear of loss of the baby and even her own life. This particularly applied to the woman having an emergency caesarean. For many of the mothers in this study, this would have been their first feeling of having a brush with *mortality*.

Clement's respondents also felt that their relationships with their babies had been damaged due to the *interruption* by, for example, general anaesthesia. This damage extended to doubts about whose baby she was caring for. Some of Clement's informants perceived that the caesarean had adversely affected their *identity*. For this woman there was a conviction that she had failed to achieve what may be regarded as the basic female function of giving birth. Thus, the woman's feelings about herself as a woman had been damaged. In slightly more concrete terms the women reported that their *body image* had been spoiled by the surgery. Words such as 'mutilated', 'butchered' or 'a piece of meat' were used to recount the woman's feelings of having been violated.

Clement's findings resonate powerfully with grief theory. Unsurprisingly, therefore, the last of the themes which she identifies is *anger*. Whereas, in grief, this tends to be unfocused, Clement found that the anger is directed largely at those whose role is supposedly to provide care. Such anger is particularly likely if the woman is unaware or uncertain of the reason for the caesarean or if she perceives that it was not genuinely necessary. It is likely that, if the woman is experiencing any distress, it is likely to be aggravated by those near to her who adopt an attitude and recite the mantra of 'Aren't you lucky . . .' Such banalities would serve only to compound the woman's feelings of distress and frustration by preventing her from articulating them.

7.1.3 Incontinence

The difficulties which women may encounter in maintaining control of their urinary and faecal/anal function after the birth have attracted much research and media attention. Whether this attention is entirely justified is difficult to assess; as is demonstrated in an account of pelvic floor damage and resulting symptoms by an oddly named 'Director of Continence' (Logan, 2005). Heavy reliance is placed on the questionable research by Sultan (1993; 1996) and Al-Mufti (1996) and their respective colleagues. The research by the Sultan group involved a sample of women who were prepared to undergo otherwise unnecessary anal investigations. The Al-Mufti work was reported in a letter, perhaps to avoid being subjected to peer review as an article would have been. The obstetricians in the Al-Mufti sample (please see section 5.4.4) were quoted as harbouring particular concerns about incontinence, on the basis of which, perhaps predictably, a more liberal attitude to caesarean was advocated.

7.1.3.1   Urinary incontinence

It is estimated that about one quarter of childbearing women experience incontinence of urine after the birth (Glazener et al, 2005). This is correctly regarded as a sizeable proportion of healthy young women with what is, at least, a socially inconvenient condition. As mentioned already, urinary incontinence is widely regarded as a direct result of vaginal birth, for which reason, caesarean may be recommended as the answer. This view is supported by a twin sisters study, which could only have been completed in the United States (Goldberg et al, 2005). The twin sisters study demonstrates, though, that caesarean, or even being childfree, does not provide complete protection from the development of this problem. Another point, which tends to be overlooked, is the even stronger association between urinary incontinence and obesity, as reflected in a high body mass index (BMI).

A study which was undertaken in a country where caesarean research could easily become a growth industry sheds helpful light on this confused and confusing picture. Brazilian researchers interviewed 189 menopausal women, of whom 52 per cent (n=98) had some urinary incontinence. Compared with never-pregnant women, the risk increased five times with having ever been pregnant. While the level of risk for women who had given birth vaginally was 4.28 times that of the never-pregnant women, women who had all their babies by caesarean still had a risk level 3.5 times greater than the never-pregnant. Thus, the major risk factor for urinary incontinence appears to be pregnancy itself. These researchers conclude that giving birth only by caesarean 'cannot honestly be offered as the solution' (Faundes et al, 2001:46).

Obviously, some authorities' contention that caesarean may be the panacea to prevent urinary incontinence is ill founded. Paradoxically, the possibility of caesarean-related iatrogenic damage to the urinary tract and/or urinary function deserves attention. The risk of damage to the bladder during surgery is small, but increases with successive caesareans (Jackson and Paterson-Brown, 2001). Similarly, the risk of damage to one of the ureters is small. The chance of caesarean, perhaps due to catheterisation, affecting bladder and/or urethral function does not appear to have been assessed.

7.1.3.2 Faecal/anal incontinence

This form of incontinence includes not only the involuntary loss of faeces, but also the accidental release of gas, flatus or wind. MacArthur and her colleagues (2001), in an international multicentre study, found that 9.6 per cent of parous women had experienced some faecal incontinence, whereas 45.3 per cent reported the unintentional loss of flatus. These researchers admit that the women's urinary function was their main focus, so the data may not be complete. The likelihood of anal incontinence was found to be marginally reduced by caesarean compared with a spontaneous birth. Far more significant, though, was the almost doubled risk of such incontinence following a birth assisted with forceps.

In the guideline developed by NICE (2004), though, the picture is shown to be even more confusing. Studies are reported which show no difference between caesarean and spontaneous births, as well as studies showing no incontinence among caesarean mothers compared with an incontinence rate of up to 23 per cent among women with vaginal births. I venture to suggest that, on the basis of these data, Al-Mufti's recommendation may, to say the least, have been somewhat premature.

7.1.4 Sexual function

The continence problems mentioned already (section 7.1.3) may be assumed to be largely or at least partly associated with pelvic floor damage sustained during vaginal birth. The extent to which such a direct link is the cause of changes in sexual functioning is even more difficult to assess. There is a widespread assumption that caesarean serves to protect the pelvic floor and facilitate more satisfactory sexual function (Barrett and McCandlish, 2002). This assumption is thought to be supported by certain celebrities' choice of giving birth by caesarean. Whereas assumption, perception and innuendo pervade our understanding of this topic, the research evidence is seriously thin.

An example of this deficiency is the oft-quoted publication by Al-Mufti and colleagues (1996), which in reality is nothing more than a letter. Particularly newsworthy was their finding that 80 per cent of the obstetrician respondents, who said they would seek a caesarean, would do so through fear of perineal damage. Equally salacious was the finding that 58 per cent of those opting for caesarean gave as their reason fear of long-term harm to their sex lives.

It is hardly surprising that the less titillating research evidence which casts doubt on the Al-Mufti findings, has not attracted the same level of media attention. For example, Hicks and colleagues in the USA highlighted the association between vaginal birth assisted with instruments and sexual dysfunction (2004). In England, however, Barrett and her colleagues undertook a more authoritative cross-sectional study involving 796 first time mothers (2005). The women were asked to recall any previous sexual problems and data were also collected on the women's attempts to resume their sexual relationship postnatally. These researchers found that there was a significant correlation between the type of birth and the couple's sexual problems in the three months after the birth. By six months, however, any persistent differences between the types of birth were too small to be significant. The only perceptible 'benefit' of caesarean in this context would seem to be in comparison with a vaginal birth assisted by forceps.

Thus, it would appear that the claims that a benefit of caesarean is that it keeps the vagina 'honeymoon fresh', may be founded more on the obstetricians' wishful thinking, rather than on any research evidence (Kenny, 2001). Any nagging questions about who is the object of such claims of 'freshness' or who is expected to benefit remain unanswered. There is a lurking suspicion that the beneficiary may not be the childbearing woman. The available research evidence has concentrated on the woman's pelvic floor and perineal function. It should not need to be stated, though, that there are many other aspects to a satisfactory sexual experience than just the movements and mechanics. It may be argued that more research attention needs to be given to the woman's self-perception and comfort with her own body and its functioning, in order to understand the resumption of sexual relations after the birth.

7.1.5 Future childbearing

A phenomenon which may not be totally unrelated to the couple's resumption of sexual activity is the likelihood of another pregnancy. A major caesarean-related factor for any future pregnancy emerged from pioneering research by Hemminki (1986), which had previously been published in a more general form with her colleagues (1985). This factor was the lower fertility after caesarean, compared with women giving birth vaginally, the reason for which has been much sought after. Since Hemminki identified this reduction in fertility following a caesarean, the finding has been endorsed elsewhere.

Of particular importance is the prospective cohort-based study by Mollison and her colleagues in Aberdeen (2005). This group of epidemiological researchers used the local database for which Aberdeen is well recognised. The study found that women who give birth by caesarean are least likely to embark on a subsequent pregnancy when compared with women whose birth is spontaneous or assisted by forceps. Further, not only is caesarean associated with a future pregnancy being less likely, it also takes longer for the woman/couple to achieve a conception. For a large proportion of the women (69 per cent, n=488) who did not embark on another pregnancy, this was through voluntary infertility. The decision to forego another pregnancy was usually related to the woman's previous experience of childbirth.

This reduction in fertility has previously been attributed to physical health problems, such as pelvic infection or surgical adhesions (Hemminki et al, 1985; Murphy et al, 2002). The causation, however, may not be as simple as these researchers suggest. Porter and her colleagues maintain that there are factors which confound this straightforward argument (2003). One of these confounders is the woman's emotional response to the caesarean (see 7.1.2) which may serve as a deterrent to further childbearing and, thus, predispose to voluntary secondary infertility. A second possible confounding factor is the persistent effect of primary infertility. This is relevant because women who were infertile before first conceiving are more likely, for a variety of reasons, to give birth by caesarean. This rationale, though, is able to explain only partly the lower post-caesarean fertility rates. Collecting data on this topic is obviously fraught with difficulties, because women who, for whatever reason, do not become pregnant again are not able to be included in the figures collected by the maternity services.

7.1.5.1 Placental development

If the woman who has previously undergone a caesarean does manage to become pregnant again, her problems are far from over. These problems relate, in the first place, to the development of the placenta. They seem to have been first highlighted by more landmark work by Hemminki, this time with Merilainen (1996). Using epidemiological techniques, these researchers were able to identify that placental development appears to be jeopardised following caresarean. The outcome of the pregnancy varies considerably with each of these problems but, almost invariably, the mother's health is put at risk, particularly through the increased likelihood of serious haemorrhage.

7.1.5.1.1 THE PATHOLOGY

Ectopic pregnancy and miscarriage – These forms of loss obviously bring to an end the current pregnancy. The risk of haemorrhage and tubal damage, caused by ectopic pregnancy, means that there are serious adverse implications for both the woman's life and for her future childbearing. Hemminki and Merilainen found that women who had previously given birth by caesarean were at greater risk of ectopic pregnancy and miscarriage, but that the difference from non-caesarean mothers was barely significant. These authors argue that, although the statistical significance is 'modest', because of the serious complications of ectopic pregnancy, these differences are 'clinically important' (1996:1573). Similarly, the data collected by Mollison and colleagues in Aberdeen (2005) appear to suggest that ectopic pregnancy is a greater risk following caesarean.

Placenta accreta – Due to the abnormal development of the feto-maternal tissues, the chorionic villi of the placenta attach themselves to the myometrial or muscle layer of the uterus, rather than just the endometrial uterine lining. Even though the placenta is able to function perfectly adequately during pregnancy, the mechanisms which facilitate separation during the third stage of labour fail to operate. This condition carries the risk of severe haemorrhage and the possible need for manual removal of the placenta or even hysterectomy (Gielchinsky et al, 2002; Höpker et al, 2002). The incidence of this condition is reported as occurring as infrequently as 1 in 93,000 pregnancies. In the series reported by Gielchinsky and colleagues, previous caesarean was a significant risk factor for placenta accreta.

Placenta percreta – This is an even less common, but more severe, form of placental maldevelopment. In this condition, the chorionic villi penetrate through the uterine wall, and adjacent organs are affected. Thus, the third stage risks of placenta accreta are further compounded. These additional risks feature damage to the other organs, such as the bladder or bowel (Gielchinsky et al, 2002).

Placenta praevia – The low-lying placenta causes difficulties with the birth as well as the risk of serious maternal haemorrhage. The research by Hemminki and Merilainen showed that first time mothers who gave birth by caesarean are at increased risk of placenta praevia in any subsequent pregnancies. In a Saudi research project, Zaki and her colleagues showed that in a series of 23,000 births, there were 100 cases of placenta praevia. Of these, in 12 women the placenta was also accreta (Zaki et al, 1998).

7.1.5.1.2 THE CAUSES

The causes of these abnormal forms of placental development are not clear. There is a possibility that placenta accreta or percreta may be due to a genetic condition which interferes with the healthy formation of the tissues underlying the placenta. Another possible mechanism, though, is that the endometrium, into which the developing placenta must embed, may have been affected in some way by previous unrecognised and untreated infection (Gielchinsky et al, 2002). A further possible explanation is that the endometrium may have been damaged by previous trauma such as during dilatation and curettage (D&C) or caesarean (Höpker et al, 2002). This possibility is considered to be most likely, particularly taking account of the greater risks associated with previous elective caesarean (Maymon et al, 2004).

While these conditions are certainly not common, as mentioned already, the risks are considerable. Because of their rarity, the incidence is uncertain. Based on published series, the incidence is thought to be low but increasing. One is left with the question, though, of how many cases do not reach the stage of being counted or published?

7.1.5.2 *The next birth*

The old maxim 'Once a caesarean – always a caesarean' is now being widely challenged through a movement which has become known as 'VBAC' (vaginal birth after caesarean). The persistence of the 'always a caesarean' attitude, though, is reflected in the widespread continuing use of a number of terms; these include 'repeat caesarean', 'secondary caesarean' or the indication for another operative birth being 'previous caesarean'. The issues informing the decisions about the mode of the next birth and the effects are addressed in detail in Chapter 8.

In most of the research literature focusing on VBAC, the outcomes are compared with elective caesarean. An important study by an Australian group, however, adopted a somewhat different approach (Taylor et al, 2005). In a novel research design, this group addressed comparisons, not according to the type of subsequent birth, but according to the type of previous birth. Thus, women who gave birth by caesarean in their last birth were compared with women whose last birth was by the vaginal route. These researchers, unsurprisingly, found that the 'previous caesarean' group were less likely to have their labour either induced or augmented. Of particular interest in these data is the finding that, among the 'previous caesarean' mothers who subsequently gave birth vaginally there was a significant increase in the number who experienced a post-partum haemorrhage (8.7 per cent compared with 5.8 per cent, n=136,101). The number who encountered complications of this haemorrhage was similarly greater. An even more disconcerting finding is that the stillbirth rate is significantly higher among the previous caesarean group (0.465 per cent compared with 0.419 per cent).

Taylor and colleagues make no attempt to explain the reasons for these differences. The authors do conclude, though, that women seeking 'an elective caesarean section for non-medical reasons in their first pregnancy should be advised of the possible consequences for their next pregnancy' (Taylor et al, 2005:517). It may be argued that presenting such data when the birthing decision is being made, which may be when the woman is in an advanced stage of labour, may be rather late. I would propose that this information should be made available to the woman at a far earlier stage in her childbearing decision making. In this way, she would be more fully aware of her choices and any potential for adverse outcomes.

7.2 Implications for the baby

As has been mentioned above (see section 7.1.5.2) an Australian study has identified the potential for increased perinatal mortality in a birth subsequent to a caesarean (Taylor et al, 2005). Thus, the supposed reduced risk to one sibling jeopardises the health and well-being of another, younger sibling. It is necessary to consider, though, whether the risks to the older sibling are actually reduced, or whether one set of immediate or short-term risks are simply replaced by another set of longer-term 'challenges' which are possibly visited on a younger sibling.

The Australian research endorsed the findings of a systematic review of pregnancy after caesarean (Hemminki, 1996). As well as the now well-recognised infertility, Hemminki showed that children born subsequently were significantly more likely to be born low birth weight (LBW) and to be vulnerable to perinatal death and to congenital malformations.

An apparently unexpected benefit resulting from changes in care in labour was observed in a Jordanian hospital (Ziadeh and Sunna, 1995). These clinicians introduced a range of changes, which over a period of seven years almost halved the caesarean rate from 15.5 per cent to 8.7 per cent. At the same time, and without any other obvious cause, the perinatal mortality rate fell even more dramatically, from 52 per 1,000 to 20.9 per 1,000. While quoting research in Sweden, Ireland, the USA and the UK showing that lowering the caesarean rate does not jeopardise the welfare of the baby, these authors are reluctant to cast any doubt on the benefits of caesarean for the baby's health.

As well as the physical health and well-being of the baby and siblings, the psychosocial outcomes deserve attention. This is particularly important in view of the effects of the mother–child relationship on the young person's development (Leitch, 1999). A comprehensive meta-analysis of English language publications focusing on psychosocial aspects of caesarean birth was undertaken by DiMatteo and her colleagues (1996). This research project showed the extent to which the baby born by caesarean misses out on the attachment-forming activities with her mother. The early mother–infant interaction in the maternity unit, as has been mentioned already (see section 6.1.2.4) is significantly reduced. DiMatteo and colleagues found that the mother later seeks to over-compensate for this initial lack.

Particularly disconcerting was the finding in this meta-analysis that caesarean mothers 'evaluate their babies less positively and have less positive feelings for them' (DiMatteo et al, 1996:305). The mother's infant feeding decision corresponds with these feelings, as babies born by caesarean are significantly less likely to be breast fed. The precise mechanism of this correspondence was not explained by these authors. It may be that both are due to the caesarean mother's relative incapacity, rather than this mother being less caring about her baby's nourishment and welfare. The mother's less positive feelings about her baby persist for at least six weeks, which has a knock-on effect on her interaction with her baby for about five months. A Scottish study endorses these findings, as Hillan found that the caesarean mothers took significantly longer to come to feel close to their babies (1992b).

The duration of these caesarean-related effects is not easy to determine. They have largely disappeared by the time the child reaches school age. In spite of this, there tend to be higher expectations of the child's performance at school for children born by caesarean. The child, as well as the parents, have been found to harbour these higher expectations (Entwistle and Alexander, 1987).

Clement (2001) is reluctant to interpret these findings as meaning that the caesarean exerts an adverse effect on the mother–child relationship. She concludes that the findings are ambiguous, examples being that the baby born by caesarean is likely to benefit in some ways, such as being given more kisses, and suffer in others, such as getting less eye contact.

There is one other psychosocial aspect which does not yet seem to have appeared in the literature and which may yet need to be considered. This relates to the parents' increased risk of infertility after a caesarean birth (see section 7.1.5 above; Mollison et al, 2005). It may be necessary to consider the position of the child born by caesarean who has no siblings. There has long been anecdotal evidence of the miserable existence of the 'only child' because of this supposed deficit. Due to the iniquitous 'one child policy' in the People's Republic of China, research into the mental health problems of the 'only child' is developing into a growth industry (Liu et al, 2005). The 'only child' in the West is also being shown to have personality difficulties (Kemppainen et al, 2001). With increasing numbers of caesareans, the 'only child' and any related difficulties, appears to be set to become more frequent.

7.3 Implications for others

So far in this chapter, we have considered the longer-term implications of caesarean for those directly involved, by this I mean the mother and baby. There may be repercussions, also, for those others who are less directly involved. These implications deserve careful attention too.

7.3.1 The father

The presence of the father in labour and at the birth has become *de rigueur* to the point of being routine. This is happening to such an extent that his being there may even be espoused by politicians (Tempest, 2006). The reasons for the father's presence is not necessarily because of any benefit to the childbearing woman (Mander, 2004a). Perhaps as a result of the general expectation of his being there, in the context of caesarean, either his presence (Inch, 1986) or his absence (Koppel and Kaiser, 2001) may prove traumatic for him (see section 3.3.3). In the period after a caesarean, it is necessary for the father to begin to come to terms with his own reaction to the birth. At the same time, he is required to adjust to becoming a father, as well as to support his partner and their child, who are recovering from surgery. It is unfortunate that the father's ability to complete all these tasks simultaneously has attracted minimal research attention. This is an omission which, for the sake of all involved, needs to be addressed as a matter of priority.

7.3.2 The care providers

Those who work in the maternity area invest in their practice to varying extents. Thus, it is necessary to explore whether and how the increasing number of caesareans is likely to affect these people. There is also the possibility of implications for their professional relationships with each other. Thus, the care providers need attention.

7.3.2.1 Implications for the midwife

The practice of the midwife is clearly changing. In considering these changes, deciding what is the cause and what the effect is certainly not easy. The midwife's changing role may be put down to organisational aspects such as the move of birth away from the home into the hospital. Alternatively, this role change may be attributed to aspects of the midwife herself, such as her education. The wide range of factors which influence midwifery practice are summarised by de Vries in terms of Geography, Technology, Societal structure, Culture (1993:133).

7.3.2.1.1 TECHNOLOGY

In the present context, it is the effect of technology which has serious repercussions for the future of midwifery, as identified by de Vries in his classic paper (1993).

De Vries discusses the ways in which the increasing use of technology serves to diminish the midwife. One of these diminutions is through the redefinition of childbirth as a health problem 'which is only normal in retrospect' and, thus, putting it in need of close medical surveillance. Obviously, such a level of *medical* supervision is outwith the midwife's scope of practice. Thus, this redefinition of childbirth means that the midwife is in danger of 'being defined out of existence' (Kirkham, 1986).

Because healthy childbearing is so closely bound up with the local culture, the transferability of midwifery expertise is limited. For this reason, the exchange or sharing of midwifery skills between different cultural groups has tended not to happen. These cultural and geographical limitations have served to constrain the midwife's global functioning. They have also weakened her position in relation to those professions which are less 'culture-bound' and whose role may overlap with hers.

De Vries continues his analysis by highlighting the importance of risk in maintaining the status of the various occupational groups who offer care to the childbearing woman. His definition of risk comprises the one used by those with a vested interest in presenting childbearing as 'high risk'. The classical professions have secured their power base by creating or emphasising the risks to which, they maintain, potential clients are exposed. Those professionals claim to have a monopoly over the ability to deliver the person from these risks. The role of the church, quoted by de Vries (1993:171), is the quintessential example of the creation of such a problem and then the offer of delivery from it. Largely with her own making or acquiescence, the midwife has removed herself or been removed from being in a position to create or emphasise risk. This is because of her staunch orientation to childbearing as a form of 'normality'. Thus, it may be that by her firm adherence to salutogenesis and to healthy childbearing, the midwife may have done herself no favours. In fact she has effectively 'shot herself in the foot'.

7.3.2.1.2 THE MIDWIFE'S RESPONSE

The crucial orientation to risk, outlined by de Vries, is endorsed by Green's research (2005). Her work demonstrates the ambivalence with which her midwife respondents viewed the risks which they encountered in their practice. The risks of childbearing were regarded as being inseparable from the threat of the ensuing litigation in the event of an adverse outcome ensuing. Thus, defensive midwifery leads the midwife to err on the side of caution. She adopts the medical strategy of assuming a 'just in case' or an 'as if' approach to her practice. Green found that the midwives she interviewed were comfortable with the rising caesarean rates. They reported feeling that there is 'too much unnecessary concern over the issue' (2005:295). Images spring to mind of ostrich-like postures and of stable doors banging shut too late.

The midwife who adopts such a *laissez-faire* attitude has been censured by Warwick (2001); she maintains that responsibility for rising caesarean rates cannot and should not be shrugged off onto obstetricians. The midwife's slightly schizoid attitudes to caesarean emerge in Warwick's paper, though. While anticipating that more home births may contribute to a resolution, Warwick concludes with a recommendation of multidisciplinary working. It may be suggested, though, that team working is actually more a part of the problem, than it is a solution.

In her consideration of 'When the midwife misses out', Inch adopts an appropriately pessimistic view of the midwife's position (1986). Although she focuses on the individual midwife, Inch's astute analysis may be no less pertinent to the midwifery profession as a whole. This doomsday scenario contemplates the de-skilling of the midwife, to the extent that she is competent only to attend women who are experiencing the most straightforward of 'normal' births. The midwife is shown to be willing, when necessary, to dispense with her midwifery attributes. Her ability, chameleon like, to assume the role of the nurse is both highlighted and deprecated. Thus, Inch's implicit message is that the rise in caesarean rates is little short of inexorable. Further, the midwife may be at risk of losing the skills even to influence the progress of labour in order to ensure a 'normal' outcome. In the event of a birth outcome which is something other than what was hoped for, Inch draws attention to the 'joint regret' (1986:67). Although such regret is shared by both the midwife and the woman, it is so profound that it is likely to remain unspoken. Thus, the two find themselves unable to unite and each remains isolated in her 'powerlessness . . . to do anything about it' (1986:67). Although Inch concludes with a vaguely optimistic suggestion that this scenario will not materialise, her Cassandra-like words appear to be starting to come true, even within the twenty years since they were published.

7.3.2.1.3 ROLE EXPANSION OR EXTENSION?

Inch's reference (above) to the midwife's role is linked to a number of changes. One of these is that, during the twentieth century, a nursing qualification became virtually mandatory for the midwife working in the UK health service. This may be the reason why she has been so willing and able to 'fill in' and perform a variety of roles which certainly do not match the definition of a midwife (ICM, 2005). This 'filling in' has included working in the operating theatre for caesareans, when the midwife has 'taken the baby', or has acted as 'runner' or has 'scrubbed'. Developments in both the UK and the US are now seeking to formalise and enlarge the midwife's role in the operating theatre. Further, attempts are afoot to build on this improvisation to establish it as a formal career path for the midwife.

Another change is that, in the UK, the European Working Time Directive (EWTD, 2003) has required managers to rethink staffing arrangements in order to achieve compliance. For some managers this rethink has involved the substitution of non-medical personnel to undertake traditionally medical functions. One example of this substitution involves the midwife acting as the assistant to the obstetric surgeon for caesareans. According to Ramsay and Paine (1997), the midwife's role is being 'extended' in order to take on work previously carried out by general practitioner trainee senior house officers. Similar arrangements have been documented in the USA; the overwhelming nursing orientation of American certified nurse-midwives (CNMs) has facilitated these developments (Moes and Thacher, 2001). The origins of the CNM acting as 'first assistant' there is somewhat different, though, in that nurses initially acted as stand-ins only in emergencies.

Such labourforce manipulations are cited as being an example of the development of the role of the midwife. Moes and Thacher seek to present this development as a form of role expansion, a concept that has been defined as: 'any enlargement of the [health care provider's] role within the boundaries of [her] education, theory and practice' (Magennis et al, 1999:33).

Role expansion is clearly a healthy and positive development in the person's career trajectory. Whether the claim of these American authors is justified, though, is quite a different matter. I would argue that the midwife, through assuming the responsibility of a house officer (a very junior medical training grade), is effectively acquiescing to her own demotion. While some may perceive any medical role as an enhancement of the status of the midwife, such a hierarchical view of health care is antediluvian. This American development might possibly be excused on the grounds of continuity of care, but this concept does not feature. The midwife in this situation is effectively being demoted to adopt the role of a 'physician extender', a term which carries highly appropriate connotations of a ventriloquist's dummy. An alternative comparison, which has been mentioned already (please see section 5.2.1.5) is with the 'medwife'.

Another way of looking at this 'development' of the midwife's role is found in the account by Ramsay and Paine in England. The medically oriented account correctly identifies these changes as role extension, defined as: 'the performance of any activities by the [health care provider] that were previously undertaken by medical doctors, or other healthcare professionals' (Magennis et al, 1999:33).

Thus, role extension is little more than substitution of a more powerful health provider with a less powerful one. There is no consideration of the individual's personal career development or of the unique qualities of their occupational group. As with so many medical tasks which some midwives have enthusiastically embraced, such as ultrasound examinations, perineal repair and epidural top-ups, the question arises of who is left to do the midwifery if the midwife is doing medical tasks? The answer is, presumably, less qualified and even less powerful personnel.

Clearly, the use of the midwife as a substitute for training grade medical staff during caesarean operations raises important questions about the function of the midwife and the organisation of health care.

7.3.2.2 Implications for the medical practitioner

The crucial role of the obstetrician in the increasing caesarean rate should not be underestimated. This role becomes particularly clear in the examination of the international situation and the close positive correlation between caesarean rates and private medical practice; although the international picture also illuminates the obstetrician's contribution (see Chapter 4). More detailed attention is given to the position of medical personnel *vis à vis* caesarean in the concluding chapter (Chapter 9).

7.4 Consumer groups

The fact that most childbearing women are young and healthy means that there is the potential for a lively interaction between the consumers and the providers of maternity services. The extent to which this interaction comes to fruition depends largely on the local culture and the health care system. The New Zealand experience is an excellent example of the success of such an interaction (Fleming, 2000). At least since the early twentieth century, when New Zealand claims to have been the first country to have given women the vote, women's rights have been fundamentally important there. The power of women manifested itself in the latter part of the twentieth century in response to the increasing medicalisation and centralisation of childbearing. A group of women consumers joined with 'one or two midwives' (Fleming, 2000:195) to ensure the woman's right to choose the place of birth. This 'Homebirth Association' was adept at publicising the debate. It was soon accompanied by another consumer group with a slightly different agenda, 'The Save the Midwives Association'. These two associations were politically astute and energetically active, demonstrating the power of the consumer, with only a little support from professionals. With this influential backing, the position of the midwife was strengthened, leading to the establishment of the New Zealand College of Midwives (NZCOM). This organisation's guiding principle is 'partnership' between women and midwives. The concept of partnership is said to operate at both an organisational as well as a personal or clinical level. The fulmination of this activity was the passage of the Nurses Amendment Act in 1990, which permitted the midwife to practise independent of any medical practitioners. As Fleming (2000) correctly identifies, the support of the then Minister of Health, Helen Clark, was crucial to the successful enactment of this legislation.

A more longstanding example of a consumer group is 'Childbearing Connection', which was founded in New York City in 1918. At that time, its name was the 'Maternity Center Association'. Its existence has been beset with threats, many due to medical practitioners who feared that competition would cause their practice and their income to decline (Lubic, 1979). Consumer groups' activities may also be threatened from within. Such threats are due to the groups' relatively informal nature and the differing priorities of the members. Thus, groups' existence tends to be discontinuous. Such groups wax and wane, form, disband and re-form according to both internal and external factors (Kitzinger, 1990).

The advent of the internet has certainly facilitated consumer groups' publicity, recruitment and general functioning (Goer, 2004). For those organisations which do not have access to this technology, however, this lack is perceived as a major impediment. Goer suggests that the stronger position of campaigning organisations since 1994 is largely attributable to the web. The creation of a group is invariably in response to the failure of some aspect of the health care service. This failure may comprise a low standard of care or a neglect of the needs of certain groups of women, such as those who are less able to argue their position.

ICAN (International Cesarean Awareness Network) is a particularly relevant example of a consumer group, having been originally entitled the 'Cesarean

Prevention Movement' when it was formed in 1982. The stimulus to its formation was the personal childbearing experience of Esther Booth Zorn. ICAN claims to have both initiated the VBAC movement and increased the availability of VBAC (ICAN, 2006). In spite of its 'International' orientation as reflected in its title, ICAN's activities are confined to the American Continent. The details of the activities of a consumer group such as ICAN are analysed by Aaronson (1991), who examined the functioning of a Women's Health Collective in ensuring the success of Rhode Island midwifery practices. As mentioned already in the New Zealand context, Aaronson identifies the political manoeuvring necessary to mount a successful campaign. Equally demonstrated in New Zealand, she emphasises the importance of the creation of a robust coalition. The purpose of this coalition is to target the stakeholders who will determine the success or otherwise of the campaign.

The role of campaigning consumer groups is clearly important in the USA and New Zealand, where single-issue groups appear to flourish. In the UK, however, such single-issue groups tend to be less common than those with a wider-ranging remit. The Association for the Improvement in Maternity Services (AIMS) is an excellent example, and the campaigning role of the National Childbirth Trust (NCT) should not be forgotten among its multiplicity of other activities (NCT, 2003).

The limited number of single-issue and campaigning groups in the UK, however, is more than compensated for by the number of post-caesarean groups offering support. This arrangement may appear to have an Alice in Wonderland quality about it. The support groups are available to help women who have been through this experience. There appears, however, to be little interest in preventing the experience that the existence of these groups appears to indicate is less than satisfactory. Although a recent search suggests that there is a multitude of post-caesarean groups with websites, Lowdon (1995b) reports the 'overwhelming apathy' that the idea of such groups generates. It may be that Lowdon's sterling work has overcome the apathy which she identified. The warning that 'support' in combination with 'caesarean' may convert this mother into a victim should be heard by all who are involved with her.

7.5 Conclusion

Some might be forgiven for envisaging the caesarean operation as a panacea. It is all too often presented as a latter day magic bullet which prevents or cures a multiplicity of childbearing problems. In this chapter I have attempted to consider the extent to which this representation is accurate. It is necessary to conclude that, while caesarean may resolve some childbearing-associated problems, it does bring with it some other implications. These implications have been shown to affect not only the childbearing woman but also those near to and around her.

Although many of the reproductive problems prevented by caesarean have been well researched, there is another area which has not been well addressed. This area is the long-term implications of caesarean which are not associated with childbearing. These areas have been subjected to little research attention. Thus, the more general aspects of the woman's life after caesarean are in urgent need of systematic study. Only in this way will it be possible to ascertain the nature of the wide-ranging long-term effects of this operation.

8   The significance of trial of labour and VBAC (vaginal birth after caesarean)

The subsequent birth after a caesarean, if there is one, raises a number of significant issues. These relate particularly to the mode or route of that birth, which may involve a trial of labour and a vaginal birth (VBAC). A number of different actors have expressed a serious interest in this subsequent birth and for a number of different reasons. In this chapter, I consider the significance of these issues to the various interested parties. This consideration begins with the historical background. The origins, particularly of VBAC, are linked with women's issues, so these are addressed then. Two research-related issues are next and are followed by four crucial health matters, ending with the all-important question of safety.

8.1 Words and the woman

8.1.1 The significance of the words

The origins and use of different terms for the subsequent birth requires attention. These origins bring with them meanings which may be less than helpful. One example is VBAC (vaginal birth after caesarean, sometimes pronounced 'vee-back'), the origins of which, like so many aspects of the caesarean story, are shrouded in mists of myth. A particularly important myth in the context of VBAC is the dictum 'once a caesarean always a caesarean'. While this dogma is generally interpreted as encouraging repeat and secondary caesareans, this was certainly not the author's original meaning. Many who have recited the mantra 'Once a caesarean . . .' cannot have realised, though, that they are both misquoting and misinterpreting what was written. Far from encouraging obstetricians to perform more caesareans, the intention of this much-maligned statement was to warn them not to undertake that first one, because of the appalling risks. In 1916, when the American obstetrician, Craigin, wrote these much-quoted words, there was another decade to pass before the technique of making the incision into the lower uterine segment would be introduced by Kerr (Flamm, 2001a). The operation which was being performed at the time Craigin was writing involved the classical or vertical uterine incision. This technique meant that the risks of uterine rupture in a subsequent pregnancy were immense; being approximately ten times greater than with the later lower segment incision. Because of these immense risks, Craigin was emphasising to

his obstetrician readers that there were long-term implications inherent in performing a woman's first caesarean. He was warning them to contemplate the risks
to the woman's life of repeated caesareans, using the following words:

> One thing must always be borne in mind, viz., that no matter how carefully a
> uterine incision is sutured, we can never be certain that the cicatrized uterine
> wall will stand a subsequent pregnancy and labor without rupture. This means
> that the usual rule is, *once a Caesarean always a Caesarean.*
>
> (Craigin, 1916:2, italics in the original)

In spite of Craigin's timely warning, and perhaps because of Kerr's innovative
incision, the enthusiasm for caesarean among their obstetric colleagues continued
to increase unabated. One result was that, fifty years later, Craigin was being
misinterpreted by an Australian obstetrician to differentiate between American
conservatism and other countries' more flexible approach: 'In the USA in general
the dictum "once a Caesarean always a Caesarean" holds' (Llewellyn-Jones,
1969:353). Whereas elsewhere 'vaginal delivery is permitted if the indication is
not recurrent' (1969:353). Llewellyn-Jones then goes on to define the clinical setting
in which this vaginal delivery after a trial of labour would be 'permitted'. A 'trial
of labour' (TOL) or trial of labour after caesarean (TOLAC) has been defined as:
'a purposeful attempt to permit active labor development with progression to
vaginal delivery' (Harer, 2002:2627).

In the case of a woman who has had a previous caesarean, it is the integrity or
strength of the uterine scar which is actually 'on trial'. There is sometimes the
impression, though, that it is the woman herself who is 'in the dock', especially
when her medical attendants refer to her as 'the candidate' (ACOG, 1999). Because
of the crucial matter of the scar in this clinical situation, this labour may be dubbed
'a trial of scar' (Flamm 2001b; Lowdon and Derrick, 2002). Unlike the former veto,
lip service now tends to be paid to the desirability of the woman with a previous
caesarean giving birth vaginally. In order for her to achieve this, though, she is
likely to be required to endure the tribulations of a 'trial of labour'. This is a labour
which, ideally, begins spontaneously. Further, medical practitioners would require
it to take place in a maternity unit providing a technologically high standard of care.
The reason for requiring this setting is that the mother, the baby and the scar are
said to need to be monitored closely, in case one of them shows any indication
that the scar is threatening to rupture.

The name applied to this labour is sufficient to cause alarm in the woman, which
would be counterproductive to the onset of her labour. The setting and the close
monitoring are likely to further aggravate the woman's anxiety and impede the
physiological progress of labour once it has begun (Lowdon and Derrick, 2002).

The ideal outcome for a trial of labour is the spontaneous birth, which the woman
is seeking. Whether she achieves this aim, or if she gives birth vaginally with
assistance, or if another caesarean is performed depends on a range of influential
factors. These factors relate to the woman herself and to those near to her, as well
as to the environment in which she labours.

8.1.2 The significance of VBAC for the consumer movement

Unsurprisingly, the backlash to the obstetric enthusiasm for caesarean also originated in the USA. Credit for the introduction of the term VBAC (vaginal birth after caesarean) is claimed by ICAN, the US-based 'International Cesarean Awareness Network' (ICAN, 2006). As mentioned already (see section 7.4) this group's agenda was clearer in its original title, the 'Cesarean Prevention Movement' (CPM), when it was formed in 1982. The stimulus to its formation was the unfortunate personal childbearing experience of its founder, Esther Booth Zorn.

Thus, the concept which is VBAC appears to have been the consumers' knee-jerk reaction to a problem created by deeply conservative and orthodox North American obstetricians. In spite of these obscure North American origins, though, the issues surrounding VBAC have assumed international significance due to the global escalation of the caesarean rate (see Chapter 4).

While VBAC was still waiting to be introduced in North America, women elsewhere were already routinely being given the opportunity to avoid a repeat or secondary caesarean. The labour in such circumstances would now be known as a 'trial of labour', although the term was not yet being used in this situation in 1969 (Llewellyn-Jones, 1969:289).

As mentioned already, CPM deserves credit for having stimulated the VBAC debate. This consumer organisation also deserves admiration for having confronted the US medical establishment; this group of women required that their 'OB/GYN's should justify their misplaced mantra of 'once a cesarean always a cesarean'. Although it was only helped by the US insurance-led health care system which regarded VBAC as the cheap alternative (Dauphinee, 2004), these women's achievement was still no mean feat. It may be, though, that the ripples from that confrontation have engulfed and may continue to engulf women and practitioners internationally. Unfortunately, it is still not clear whether these altercations have benefited the many women who are, even now, still being denied either a trial of labour or a VBAC.

8.1.3 The significance to the woman

The meaning to the woman of making the decision about the subsequent birth may be quite straightforward. We may assume that this applies equally to deciding to give birth vaginally after a caesarean. We may be forgiven for thinking that this decision is little more than a reaction to a bad experience or the result of medically controlled information. The reality, however, has been shown to be far more complex and important.

A multiplicity of information sources is a feature of the woman's decision making in this situation (Meier and Porreco, 1982). These sources include her partner, friends, relatives and magazines, as well as a range of health care personnel. The woman's personal expectations of and aspirations for motherhood also feature prominently in her processing of the information which she obtains. Alongside the desire for a 'natural' birth experience, the woman adopts a quite pragmatic approach to the fact that there are risks to a major surgical operation such as caesarean (Fawcett et al, 1994). She also takes into account what she knows of its likely effects on her early days and months of motherhood.

A qualitative study by Ridley and her colleagues (2002), though, was able to probe deeply into the significance of deciding on a vaginal birth for this woman. The sample was a small group of women who had had a successful VBAC. The woman was found to value the sense of control which making this decision gave her. This control extended as far as locating material to counter the arguments advanced by her obstetrician. On the other hand, the woman would occasionally find that her physician would offer her good support for her VBAC decision. The woman was particularly helped by being able to locate evidence-based material detailing the beneficial outcomes of VBAC. This material contrasted markedly with some of the horror stories with which she was being bombarded from other sources. On the basis of these findings, Ridley and her colleagues conclude that the woman's decision is influenced by a range of both internal and external factors. The final decision, though, is an intensely personal one, being the product of much research and careful deliberation.

While, obviously, the decision about the subsequent birth is highly specific, there may be other unanticipated benefits to the experience of taking this decision. An example of these benefits includes the opportunity for the woman to reflect on a wide range of her own personal beliefs and values (Wickham, 2002). In order to make her childbearing decisions, Wickham encourages the woman to contemplate a number of aspects. These include her 'goals in life', where and in whom she places her trust and identifying her 'core philosophy' (2002:25).

Another not unrelated benefit emerges from the work of Lowdon and Derrick (2002). Writing particularly for consumers, these authors focus on the decisions which the woman may be required to take during her labour. The woman is encouraged 'to remain in control of the situation' (2002:7), as is shown to be important by Ridley and her colleagues. The authors go on to state that the likelihood of a successful VBAC is much higher if the woman is able to maintain this assertive outlook. The woman may be assisted in developing this outlook by the backing of others who have been through or are going through the experience of a VBAC; thus the crucial significance of 'caesarean birth meetings' starts to become apparent (Lowdon, 1995b:11).

8.2 Research matters

8.2.1 *The epidemiological significance*

The escalating caesarean rates throughout the world (see Chapter 4) have attracted appropriately massive attention and conjecture. Mainly because of the impact of this 'cesarean epidemic' (Kitzinger, 1998:56) on the health budget in the USA, ways of reducing the rates have fervently been sought. The appearance on the scene of the VBAC movement must have been welcomed like the answer to US health economists' prayers. Perhaps due to the activity of the VBAC movement, in the early 1990s the US VBAC rate almost doubled (Kozak and Weeks, 2002). The result was that approximately one third of babies born subsequently after caesareans were vaginal births. This manifested itself in a temporary reversal in the inexorable rise in the US caesarean rate from 1991.

Unfortunately, the general and professional media soon became aware of this drop in the caesarean rates. The resulting adverse publicity caused this drop to be a short-lived 'blip' (Mozurkewich and Hutton, 2000). So, from 1995, the VBAC rate itself began to decline and there was a reciprocal increase in the number of caesareans. By 2001, the US caesarean rate had not only reached, but had exceeded the levels prior to the VBAC 'blip' (Meikle et al, 2005). As is so often the case, the UK figures followed the US pattern but with a slight time lag (Black et al, 2005). It may be argued, therefore, that the current practice of VBAC may not offer the solution to the problem of the caesarean epidemic. Whether the reason for such pessimism is found in women's health or in the media industry is difficult to assess.

I venture to suggest, though, that the problem of the caesarean rates may not be amenable to such a simplistic message as that propounded by groups such as ICAN. Clearly, accurate research-based information is needed by both women and practitioners about the benefits and risks of trial of labour and VBAC (see section 8.3.2 below). It may be, though, that an approach on several fronts is necessary to address this issue, as suggested by Churchill (2003:159).

An audit of caesarean in England and Wales, examined the number of primary caesareans, which is a caesarean in a woman who has not had a caesarean previously, irrespective of her parity (Thomas and Paranjothy, 2001:20). These auditors compared this number with the secondary or repeat caesareans. They found that the repeat caesarean rate is approximately four times as high, compared with the rate for primary caesareans. This figure demonstrates that, if permitted, it would be possible to reduce the caesarean rate significantly by greater availability of VBAC.

This picture is further complicated, though, by comparison of emergency and elective caesarean rates. Of the number of primary caesareans, approximately two thirds of them are undertaken in an emergency (Thomas and Paranjothy, 2001:20). The importance of the emergency caesareans has been demonstrated in Scotland; here the rate of emergency caesareans has been found to have almost doubled since 1990; whereas the elective caesarean rate has only increased by around 40 per cent (SPCERH, 2005:22). Thus, issues of maternal choice have quite rightly been discussed in terms of their contribution to escalating caesarean rates. The contribution of emergency caesareans, though, has made a far greater difference to the incidence of caesarean, but has attracted minimal interest among the popular media.

If an attempt is to be made, therefore, to reduce the caesarean rates, an approach needs to be made on at least two fronts. The proportion of secondary caesareans may be reduced by a change of culture among women and health care providers; this would be achieved by increasing the availability and acceptability of VBAC. The number of emergency caesareans also needs to be addressed, though. It is necessary to resolve the problem, not only of the number, but also the increasing rate of emergency caesareans. Thus, what is necessary is a slowing down of the increase or a reduction in the number of emergency caesareans. Such an approach would affect not only caesarean as a public health issue, but also the implications for the individual woman, as noted by the Select Committee on Health:

> Unless the primary caesarean rate can be cut, that is reducing the number of women who have a first caesarean, the overall rate will continue to rise and women will have their opportunities for choice and control limited.
>
> (SCoH, 2003)

It is clear, therefore, that the epidemiology of trial of labour and VBAC is not only of significance to epidemiologists, but also to increasing numbers of childbearing women and those who provide care for them.

8.2.2 The significance of research

As shown already, the recognition among North American obstetricians of the feasibility of successful trial of labour and VBAC was disappointingly short-lived. The reason for the brevity of these obstetricians 'finally joining their European colleagues in offering the option of trial of labour' has been attributed to nagging concerns about rupture of the uterus (Flamm, 2001a:81). The unfortunate transience of this window of opportunity may have been an example of the effect of peer pressure superimposed on longstanding, yet ill-founded, anxieties. Medical parochialism, verging on xenophobia, was demonstrated by Enkin (1992), who has shown that it leads to distrust of widely disseminated research-based information. He emphasises the overwhelmingly powerful roles of local contacts and peer pressure in the belief systems of these medical practitioners. According to Enkin's assertions, more authoritative research regarding the risks and benefits of VBAC would have made little, if any, difference to its continuing availability. It may be suggested that these reasons underpin the widespread continuing adherence to Craigin's misinterpreted dictum (1916, please see section 8.1 above). Against this background, the significance of research *vis à vis* VBAC may be difficult to assess. The current position, though, requires close and careful scrutiny.

The medical profession has long claimed that its practice is based on 'science'; thus, practitioners claim that they are 'scientists' (Hunt, 1801). These claims have more recently undergone some revision. The 'science' has been revised, first, to encompass research-based medicine and, even more recently, as evidence-based medicine (EBM), which has been defined in the following terms: 'the conscientious, explicit and judicious use of current best evidence in making decisions about the care of individual patients' (Sackett et al, 1996:71).

The need for 'evidence' was initiated by the dreadful observations made by Cochrane in 1972. He identified and deplored the dearth of scientific rigour in clinical decision making by medical practitioners. He went on to single out obstetricians for withering criticism, because of their total lack of such rigour. Some obstetricians, together with other colleagues practising in the maternity area, have responded to this scathing condemnation, by attempting to put the obstetric house in order. The extent of their success is apparent in the caesarean-focused discussion (below).

Many column inches have been devoted in the medical media to VBAC and trial of labour/labor. Using these words as search terms, a Medline search found 1,395 publications. The quality of these publications, though, and their likely effect on practice has generally escaped scrutiny. An exception to this observation is found in the work of Dodd and Crowther in Adelaide, Australia. These researchers have long been endeavouring to make firm recommendations about the use of caesarean, trial of labour and VBAC. One recent publication in the form of a systematic review clearly shows the evidence base of medical advice to women about the subsequent birth (Dodd and Crowther, 2004a).

Using the stringent criteria appropriate to a systematic review, Dodd and Crowther were able to identify eight studies which were prospective, as opposed to utilising the less reliable retrospective data. These eight studies met the reviewers' criteria of comparing planned elective caesarean with a planned VBAC. Six of the studies, though, needed to be excluded as they introduced greater variability by including women who had had more than one caesarean, women who had previously had one successful VBAC or women who were not really suitable for VBAC. The result was that these researchers were able to identify only two studies which they considered provided useful guidance to those who had a previous caesarean and are contemplating a vaginal birth.

A major weakness of this research literature, according to Dodd and Crowther, is the absence of any studies which meet that gold standard for EBM – the randomised controlled trial (RCT). Although the strengths of RCTs are probably unarguable, it is necessary to question the feasibility of undertaking such a research project in the context of VBAC. In order to undertake an RCT, though, it would be necessary to recruit and randomise a suitable sample of childbearing women. This would involve pregnant women being given complete information about the issues, including the possible risks, of each type of birth. On the basis of this information each woman would be asked to consent to being randomised to either an intervention group (VBAC) or a control group (elective caesarean). This process would mean that the woman would have an equal chance of being in a group to have one mode of birth or the other; that is, being allocated to an elective repeat caesarean or allocated to the trial of labour group with a view to VBAC.

It is likely that, even if such a study were to be given ethical committee and managerial approval to go forward, women would have serious misgivings about being randomised. Even though women have been shown to possess a clear understanding of what is involved in randomisation, each woman's innermost feelings and concerns about one mode of birth or the other would inevitably affect the outcome. This means that if a woman preferring VBAC were to be randomised to the elective caesarean group, her displeasure and concerns might affect her recovery from her surgery. On the other hand, in the event of a woman wishing for an elective caesarean being randomised to the VBAC group, her misgivings and anxiety would be likely to affect her progress in labour. Thus, the chance of a successful VBAC would be reduced. So, for both groups of women, the process of randomisation would without doubt bring some disappointments. It goes without saying that any woman would be free to withdraw from an RCT at any point should she have any wish to do so. Clearly, though, women withdrawing from the study would inevitably reduce the value of the study findings.

In spite of these concerns, at the time of writing Dodd and Crowther are 'in the planning stage of a study related to birth after caesarean' (Dodd et al, 2004:7). It may be possible to assume that this is the RCT which these researchers have emphasised has not already been undertaken. The progress of this study will be observed with keen interest among researchers working in the field of childbearing. The findings will also be awaited by women and practitioners, as well as by others who also have an interest in trial of labour and VBAC.

Using strict criteria for their systematic review, Dodd and Crowther identify two studies which are likely to be helpful to women and practitioners. The first was a study by Iglesias and his colleagues (1991), who practised in a small (230 births per annum) community hospital in Alberta, Canada. One of the strategies used by these physicians to reduce the caesarean rate was the encouragement of trial of labour and VBAC. Over a five-year period in the late 1980s, 137 women were identified as suitable for VBAC. A large proportion (47 per cent, n=65) either declined VBAC or were not offered it, suggesting some misgivings among both the women and their health care providers. Of the remaining 72 women, 81 per cent (n=58) enjoyed a successful VBAC. It is necessary to consider that the physicians in this study may have actually managed to change the birthing culture of this community of nine thousand souls. The published data certainly indicate that the proportion of women agreeing to a trial of labour increased steadily over the five-year period. At the same time, the number of women not offered or refusing VBAC declined reciprocally. The most serious maternal problems encountered by these physicians were two cases of scar dehiscence (see section 8.3.1). These data reinforce the observation made already (see section 8.2.1), that culture change is necessary if problematical caesarean rates are to be addressed.

The other study identified by Dodd and Crowther was the one by Abitbol and colleagues in a New York City hospital (1993). These researchers report on 312 women who would have been eligible for a trial of labour. Of these women, 40 per cent (n=125) refused to participate in the VBAC programme. The reasons given for this refusal were convenience combined with fear of a repeat of a traumatic first birth. Of the 187 women who participated in the VBAC programme, 65 per cent (n=122) did give birth vaginally. About one quarter of these women, though, were not happy with their experience, stating that they would have preferred an elective caesarean. The reasons for each of the women agreeing to VBAC related to her desire for a 'natural' birth and fear of the risks of surgery for her and her baby. In this study, one woman experienced a rupture of the uterus, her baby was stillborn and she was required to undergo a hysterectomy.

These two studies identified by Dodd and Crowther demonstrate a number of useful issues. Similarly, a larger series by Mozurkewich and Hutton (2000) shows how research may be used differently. These authors report a meta-analysis of VBAC and trial of labour over the ten-year period leading up to 1999. Unlike Dodd and Crowther's, this study does not adhere to strict criteria for the selection of items. Additionally, Mozurkewich and Hutton are 'creative' in their interpretation of statistical significance and their 'innovative' classification of perinatal deaths. Disconcertingly, these researchers conclude, on the basis of these statistical manoeuvres, that the maternal outcomes and perinatal mortality are worse in trial of labour and VBAC.

Although the debate over trial of labour and VBAC has, at the time of writing, been alive and well in maternity circles for at least two decades, it seems to have engendered infinitely more heat than light. On the basis of this brief analysis, it is clear that research findings are limited. This applies to both the quantity and the quality of research. The systematic review by Dodd and her colleagues demonstrates the paucity of authoritative research evidence. On the basis of the limited number of studies and their questionable quality, these researchers warn the reader that the conclusions of the studies reviewed need to be interpreted with caution (Dodd et al, 2004:7). Whether this 'health warning' is associated in any way with these researchers' own planned study is difficult to assess.

In spite of these limitations, however, the trial of labour and VBAC rates have plummeted and allowed caesarean rates to revert to their former meteoric rise. This practice of decision making in the absence of authoritative research must cast doubt on any medical claims to either being scientific or practising evidence-based health care.

8.3 Health issues

8.3.1 The significance of healing and other processes

At this point it may be helpful, in order to better understand the significance of the issues around VBAC, to revisit the physiological processes in the surgical wound following the caesarean operation. These processes, as when any physical wound is inflicted, are fundamentally important to the successful healing of the uterine wound. Their effectiveness may also carry implications for the outcome of any future pregnancy.

In general terms, the adequacy of wound healing has been shown to be affected by a range of factors. These include the person's age, nutrition, hydration, cleanliness, freedom from infection, pharmacological treatment and tissue oxygenation (RCSE, 2006). Clearly, in a childbearing woman who, by definition, is relatively young these factors will ordinarily function healthily; thus ensuring that the wound in her uterus heals optimally and securely.

When the uterine wound heals, as happens with any other, there is a localised physiological inflammatory reaction. Platelets and thrombin in the wound form a network with the collagen fibres. Cells, such as macrophages, are carried to the wound site and fibroblasts develop to facilitate healing and the formation of a scar. In this way, the wholeness or integrity of the uterus is usually re-established.

This process is significant because, if the conditions for healing are less than ideal, it may not be completed healthily. This means that, under certain circumstances, the edges of a wound, which was thought to have healed, may begin to separate or undergo 'dehiscence'. These circumstances may include tension on the previously wounded structure. In the present context, this tension would be inevitable in a subsequent pregnancy or labour. Should the tension be sufficient to lead to separation, it would manifest itself as rupture of the uterus, about which the term 'dehiscence' is usually used to indicate a mild degree (Guise et al, 2004).

The effects of rupture of the uterus, like the extent of the rupture, vary hugely. The rupture or dehiscence may be so slight as to be asymptomatic. In this situation, neither the woman nor her attendants would be able to detect any changes to make them suspect a rupture. Thus, the rupture may only be identified if and when a caesarean is undertaken for some other reason. At the opposite end of the continuum of severity, the effects of the uterine rupture may be drastically different. Then the consequences for the mother, the baby or both may be dire. In such serious circumstances, this rupture may be referred to as 'complete' or 'true'.

Partly because of this variation in severity, the incidence of rupture of the uterus is not easy to quantify. Obviously, the milder forms may pass unnoticed and unrecorded. In an authoritative systematic review, a pooled figure emerged for all the studies reviewed of 3.8 ruptures per 1,000 women who laboured after a previous caesarean (Guise et al, 2004). When considering the incidence, though, it is necessary to bear in mind that rupture of the uterus does not only occur in women who have previously had a caesarean.

8.3.2 Trial of labour and birth outcomes

Although the term *trial* of labour carries a number of connotations which are far from woman-friendly, it is useful here because it serves to distinguish women who seek a VBAC from the relatively large proportion who are successful. This distinction matters if the woman is to be given accurate figures on which to base her decision for a subsequent birth.

The published data suggest that a woman who embarks on a trial of labour with a view to VBAC, is more than likely to be successful. In a Canadian meta-analysis over a ten-year period, 28,813 women began labour, out of 47,682 who were eligible (60 per cent) (Mozurkewich and Hutton, 2000). Of these, 20,746 women (72 per cent) successfully achieved a VBAC.

Unfortunately, the data for England and Wales are less helpful. From their audit data, Thomas and Paranjothy (2001) report that only 44 per cent of eligible women are offered a trial of labour, and that the proportion varies between 8 per cent and 90 per cent. These auditors, though, do not detail the number of women who accept this offer and go into labour. The reader is merely informed that the VBAC rate was found to be 33 per cent. If the reader surmises that all of the women who are offered a trial of labour accept this offer, then the successful VBAC rate would be 75 per cent. The fact that the 'success rate' is not provided may serve to indicate these authors' priorities.

An even more recent study, albeit in North America, provides data which are helpful to both the woman and her health care providers. Landon and his colleagues (2004) undertook a cohort study involving women attending 19 US medical centres between 1999 and 2002. There were 378,168 women in the cohort and 45,988 were eligible to give birth by VBAC. Of these women, 17,898 opted for a trial of labour (38.9 per cent) and a large majority (73.4 per cent, n=13,139) were successful in giving birth vaginally.

These data show that, although cultural and professional factors clearly influence the number of women who are able to begin a trial of labour, the success rate for women who do is both reassuringly high as well as being remarkably consistent.

8.3.3 The significance of health problems

Although it has been shown that successful VBAC is the outcome in approximately three out of four women beginning a trial of labour, the outcome for the other one in four women also needs attention.

Because it has traditionally been the major source of concern, I address uterine rupture first. The large American study (Landon et al, 2004) demonstrated that the rate of rupture of the uterus during trial of labour was 0.7 per cent (n=124/17,898). This rate is high compared with the 0.4 per cent rate found by Mozurkewich and Hutton (2000) in the data which were collected when VBAC was more popular and acceptable. Interestingly, Landon and his colleagues do not mention the incidence of rupture of the uterus in the elective caesarean group. While it may be that no women in this group experienced a rupture, this is unlikely, as other surveys have featured such occurrences. In Canada, for example, women having an elective caesarean had a rupture rate of 0.2 per cent (Mozurkewich and Hutton, 2000), while in California among these women the rupture rate was 0.3 per cent (Gregory et al, 1999).

Landon and his colleagues make only passing reference to two particularly serious maternal outcomes. They maintain that this cursory attention is because the differences were not significant, so they give little attention to the hysterectomy rate and maternal mortality rate. This is in spite, or perhaps because, of these rates having been higher in the elective caesarean group of women. The reader may be forgiven for wondering whether these authors have their own 'agenda' and whether the data are either being emphasised or played down in order to fit that agenda. These suspicions are confirmed when the perinatal risks attract a disproportionately high level of attention. The focus of the perinatal problems is the 'hypoxic–ischemic encephalopathy' developed by 12 babies following a trial of labour. The severity or functional deficits associated with this condition are not mentioned. It is necessary to wonder whether this condition is being publicised, rather like a shroud being waved, in order to alarm women contemplating VBAC. In the same way, 'neonatal seizures' have been used to persuade women to accept continuous electronic fetal monitoring (CEFM) in labour, until the absence of any long-term effects of such seizures was explained (Alfirevic et al, 2006). It is necessary to bear in mind, though, that neonatal 'hypoxic–ischemic encephalopathy' is not due directly to the trial of labour, but to the rupture of the uterus. As mentioned already, this dire outcome is not totally prevented by an elective caesarean.

Thus, it would appear that the risks to the mother of rupture of the uterus have ceased to be a major concern. This may be because the serious risks are not significantly different between women beginning a trial of labour and those opting for an elective caesarean. Medical researchers appear to have completed something of a 'U-turn' and are now threatening women with the 'greater perinatal risks' without providing any detail of their nature or significance.

8.3.4 The significance of iatrogenesis

The concept of iatrogenesis has been raised already in relation to the problems associated with caesarean (please see section 6.5). This concept, though, assumes a special significance in the context of trial of labour and VBAC (Dodd and Crowther, 2004b). The reason is that, like other women, a woman who has previously given birth by caesarean may develop a problem which requires the baby to be born before labour starts spontaneously. Examples include pre-eclampsia or poor intrauterine growth (IUGR). The picture is further complicated if the woman's pregnancy has extended past the due date and is regarded as 'post-term'.

This situation is problematical because, while the pregnancy may need to be ended and the baby born, an elective caesarean is less than ideal. The option which remains is induction of labour. The risks ordinarily inherent in induction of labour are aggravated by the presence of the woman's uterine scar. Pharmacological agents which are used to induce or accelerate labour, such as misoprostol or prostaglandin E_2 have clearly been shown to increase the risk of rupture of the uterus (Blanchette et al, 1999). The solution to this enigma, according to Wagner, is to reduce the number of inductions of labour but that, he maintains, 'is not a doctor-friendly solution' (2002:368).

8.4 The significance of safety

The safety of trial of labour and VBAC has been shown to be a source of concern, particularly, for researchers and practitioners. The extent of this concern emerges from an, admittedly cursory, literature search. By entering 'trial of labour' or 'trial of labor' and 'VBAC' into the databases CINAHL and Medline, 425 items were identified. When I added safe or safety, 73 of these items were found to address this aspect. Because of the considerable attention given to it in the professional literature, if for no other reason, the topic of safety deserves careful examination. In this section, I scrutinise the meaning of safety and attempt to assess whether it is possible for trial of labour and VBAC to be offered safely.

8.4.1 The physical safety of the woman and baby

The physical health of the woman and her baby is what is ordinarily meant when the word 'safety' is used in this context. Ensuring physical health is probably the most fundamental aim of the health care provider. This aim may have originated with the work of Hippocrates when he wrote 'Of Epidemics' in 400 BCE. Since then, this ideal has been handed down in the form of the ethical principle of beneficence or non-maleficence. This concept is summarised in the dictum *Primum non nocere* (First, do no harm), on which the Hippocratic oath is founded; although the ethical basis of that oath has been accused of being less than altruistic (Thompson et al, 2006:209). The ethical principle of non-maleficence was applied to an institutional health care setting by Florence Nightingale, when she recognised the paradox inherent in the need to even mention it: 'It may seem a strange principle to enunciate as the very first requirement in a hospital that it should do the sick no harm' (1859). These historical origins reflect the quite basic standard which physical safety represents. The discussion of iatrogenesis (see section 6.5) suggests that the achievement of even this basic standard may be beyond the reach of some health care agencies.

In the context of caesarean, it was the long-term physical safety of the woman that prompted Craigin to pen his immortal yet much maligned dictum '*once a Caesarean always a Caesarean*' (1916). In this warning to his obstetrician colleagues about the implications of performing that first caesarean, he was contemplating not only the limitation of the woman's childbearing capacity, but also the possibility of shortening her life. Since Craigin first wrote these words, the maternal outcomes have continued to drive the debate on, first, trial of labour and, later, VBAC. Only recently, perhaps due to professional and popular denial of adverse maternal outcomes, has this focus begun to change (Mander, 2001b). The focal point of the debate on the safety of trial of labour and VBAC has been shown to be moving away from the mother's safety in the direction of that of her baby (Landon et al, 2004). The rationale for this movement may only be surmised. The anxiety, though, is that it may relate to the childbearing woman's recognised tendency to prioritise the welfare of her baby over her own well-being. Thus, any argument impinging on the health of her baby is more likely to be effective in persuading her than any consideration of her own safety. The fact that the debate is now being moved in this direction should, therefore, be a source of some concern.

8.4.2 Safety/security of staff

It may be that this prioritisation of the baby's welfare is not unique to the child-bearing woman. The tendency of a range of professionals to focus on the baby's well-being, possibly at the cost of the mother's, has been dubbed 'fetocentrism' (see section 5.5). In Canada, Bassett and his colleagues identify the same phenomenon and define it as 'intense concern for the immediate and future health of the fetus' (2000:529). They label it, however, 'Doctors as fetal champions', clearly suggesting that it is they alone who have fetal health as their primary interest. These researchers argue that this orientation, a by-product of the technological advances in maternity care, is what leads to defensive practice, as opposed to any malpractice litigation. Thus, health care personnel are endeavouring to stay 'one step ahead' of litigious clients and their legal advisors; they do this by focusing all their attention on the fetus, whose welfare is everyone's 'bottom line'. In this way, staff may resort to such defensive practice in order to ensure their own safety or security.

A more traditional approach to the safety of the health care provider is advanced by Dauphinee (2004). Writing from a North American setting, she endeavours to link the safety of the 'patient' striving for a VBAC, with the nurse's safety. The only link between these two concepts is found in practising sufficiently defensively to guarantee freedom from litigation. To achieve this, Dauphinee places an over-whelming emphasis on information giving; in this way she claims to ensure that the woman understands the risks of embarking on a trial of labour. All of this information is recommended to be given both verbally and in writing before the consent form may be signed. One may be forgiven for wondering whether a woman opting for an elective caesarean would be informed of the risks so comprehensively. The major threat to the safety of a trial of labour, therefore, appears to be putting the 'nurses, physicians and hospital at risk for a lawsuit' (2004:113)

Thus, it would seem that it is the uncertainty inherent in beginning a trial of labour, with a view to VBAC, which is perceived as a threat to the safety of the staff. This safety may comprise their occupational comfort zone which may be threatened by the possibility of disciplinary action or litigation. Alternatively, the threat may be to the smooth running of the labour and delivery department by a woman seeking the birth experience which she feels is appropriate for both her and her baby.

8.4.3 Safety/security of the woman

In the institutional settings in which the vast majority of UK women give birth the staff are, effectively, on their own territory. This is where the staff are at home. They feel comfortable and are in a position to welcome the woman and encourage her to feel relaxed so that the birth can progress as it should. In spite of the staff's best efforts, though, the woman knows that she is on alien territory. As a result, her body may not allow itself to function physiologically. This scenario has been portrayed as a failure of the 'fetus ejection reflex' (Odent, 1987). It represents an example of the way in which the socio-physiological processes of labour may be inhibited by interventions which inadvertently threaten the woman's need for con-fidence in her own safety and security. In her analysis of the close interdependence between safety and trust, Kirkham endorses safety's crucial role if the woman is to achieve her 'maximum potential' (2000:242). In the present context this is the potential to complete a trial of labour culminating in VBAC. The safety to which Kirkham refers comprises a total environment in which the woman's independence is supported so well that she does not need to prove it. In such a safe environment the woman is able to allow herself to become dependent on her carers as and when she decides that it is appropriate.

This meaning of safety to the woman is further endorsed by a qualitative study of women's place of birth decision making (Edwards, 2005). This study found that, contrary to the views of professionals such as Bassett and colleagues (see section 8.4.2), there is no doubt that the woman is the one who is most concerned about the welfare of her baby and herself. Edwards showed that a crucial aspect is the woman's need to have her concerns respected, rather than refuted. Thus, to the woman, safety is a very individual phenomenon, which means much more than mere physical well-being. Further, Edwards identified the woman's need to locate midwifery support which would accept one concern in particular; that is, her anxiety about the technological aspects of birth. In this way the woman's need for safety could be met within a holistic milieu. Obviously ensuring such safety requires a supremely high standard of midwifery care, which would be built on a profoundly trusting relationship between the midwife and the woman. Edwards identified that this relationship, however, might be threatened by certain organisational developments which may prevent the midwife from practising fully autonomously. Such impediments would serve to undermine the trust between the woman and the midwife, as neither would be able to be confident of the effects of this third party on their relationship.

Thus, the way in which the woman interprets safety has been shown to be more broadly all-encompassing than the interpretation by some of her professional carers. Edwards, further, found that her informants were pragmatically realistic about the feasibility of ensuring physical safety. Each of the women in her study recognised the relative nature of safety and the limited extent to which any degree of safety can be completely assured. This is an eminently level-headed view of safety; it resonates powerfully with a midwifery view which, for obvious reasons, tends not to be articulated (Magill-Cuerden, 1997).

Safety is one of the issues addressed in a booklet on VBAC intended for the childbearing woman (Lesley, 2004). The woman's 'emotional and psychological safety' (2004:31) emerges as crucially important. One of the ways in which this woman may be recommended to achieve such safety is by a home birth (HBAC). One woman reports how coming to understand the reality of her previous surgical birth experiences encouraged her to choose to successfully give birth at home subsequently:

> I thought I was well informed. I'd read loads of books and magazines, I had a bit of nursing experience. I thought that women who homebirthed were lentil eating madwomen who carelessly put their babies' lives in danger. I wanted to be where the medical equipment was. Two caesareans later I read the evidence and realised where 'being where the evidence was' had got me.
>
> Jenny HBA3C (2004:31)

8.4.4 *The baby's voice*

In many areas of health care research the voice of the consumer is now beginning to be heard more clearly. This applies to research such as that involving people with mental health problems or learning difficulties as well as with children. It may be surprising, therefore, that the voice of the person born by caesarean is not heard.

Clearly, hearing this voice is not easy and it may take a long time. The process has been begun by Lesley Downie (2006), who has described her observations of the baby born by elective caesarean. These observations include the challenges which this baby faces, such as the physical, physiological, emotional and psychological aspects. Although such subjective observations may be criticised, they share some common ground with Leboyer's thoughts (1975). Some may recall that, although his ideas were not well received at the time, Leboyer was eventually responsible for a whole raft of sustained changes in birthing practice.

Perhaps, with the escalating caesarean rates, now would be an opportune time to begin to ascertain whether there are any differences between the baby born by caesarean and the baby born vaginally.

8.4.5 *The safety of VBAC*

On the basis of this discussion of safety of trial of labour and VBAC, the outcome is not entirely clear. Whether VBAC is able to be offered safely clearly depends on a number of factors. The main factors relate, first, to what is meant by safety and whether an absolute or a relative measure of safety is being used. It may be suggested that absolute safety at the birth is not feasible; in the same way that it cannot be assured in any aspect of human existence. The second factor relates to whose safety is being considered. It may be that the safety of one person or one group of people exerts a serious threat to the well-being of another.

8.5 Conclusion

Issues relating to trial of labour and VBAC seem to have been pushed to the sidelines by the debate around maternal choice and caesarean on request. In this chapter I have shown that the issues around the subsequent birth are too significant to allow them to be sidelined.

An issue which tends not to attract much attention is one reason why many women may be reluctant to embark on a trial of labour. The issue is fear, founded on previous experience. In a New York study the proportion of refusals was 40 per cent of the women eligible for trial of labour (Abitbol et al, 1993). The authors report that the women articulated fear of a repetition of a traumatic previous birth experience. These anxieties are due to the woman's assumption that the pattern of her previous labour is likely to repeat itself. Thus, a woman whose first labour ended with an emergency caesarean for dystocia or failure to progress is likely to anticipate that her second labour will be a rerun of the first. This assumption is likely to be reached because she thinks that the factors which determine the outcome of labour are purely physical and unaltered and unalterable. Midwives are very well aware of the multiplicity of bio-psychosocial phenomena which are likely to influence the outcome of a labour and birth. Not least amongst these phenomena is the effect of the woman's experience. This includes her experience of labour and birth by caesarean and her experience of raising a baby before conceiving again. These factors are likely to change both the woman and her subsequent childbearing experience – probably to make the labour more effective and increase the likelihood of a successful VBAC. The medical profession has for some reason not sought to disabuse the woman and other members of the public of the incorrect nature of this assumption.

9   Conclusion

In this book a number of important themes have emerged out of the research, literature and other sources. These themes relate to the meaning and implications of caesarean for the major participants in the childbearing scenario. By this, I mean the woman, her baby and those who attend her. In this conclusion I draw together these crucial themes and scrutinise their significance.

9.1 The status of caesarean

Caesarean has, since mythological times, been thought to imbue the person born in this way with exceptional powers and abilities. As I showed in Chapter 1, these abilities have extended to godliness, with caesarean having been referred to as 'the godly way to enter the world' (Trolle, 1982:9). Thus, the baby's origins were even then regarded as high status in spite, or perhaps because, of the likely demise of the mother.

More recently, though, the highly elevated status of caesarean has assumed a distinctly different meaning. This is reflected in the caesarean operation having been dubbed 'a cut above' (presumably compared with other modes of birth) (Clement, 1995:36). This is a figure of speech which may be interpreted as alluding not only to the anatomical site of the caesarean incision, but also to the status of the operation and the woman who undergoes it.

The 'superiority' of caesarean may be due to a couple of factors. First, in recent times, caesarean has been shown (see Chapter 4) to be more favoured by and easily available to the most wealthy women. This is largely due to private systems of medicine which may function independently of or in co-existence with a state funded system of health care. Second may be the moral superiority of women who have had an emergency caesarean and have had to experience both the pain of labour and the pain and other challenges of postoperative recovery. Thus, but probably for very different reasons, the status of caesarean is once again proving to be elevated.

The question of who is likely to benefit from this elevation of caesarean's status is one which, I hope, has been answered through the medium of this book. It will be enough to state here that for many of the women, apart from possibly being able to contribute to the decision, the benefits are not as great as we are sometimes led to believe. The advantages for most of the babies born by caesarean seem to be more apparent than real. Little is so far known about this father's experience; so the jury is still out on what he does or does not gain from being present at his partner's caesarean. Traditionally, the midwife has not been directly involved in the caesarean. This may be changing, though, and may have serious implications for the midwife's role (see section 7.3.2.1.3). The other party directly involved in the caesarean scenario is the medical practitioner or practitioners. The nature of their gain, especially in countries with a thriving private health sector (see Chapter 4), is all too obvious. What are the benefits to obstetricians in other settings, though? The answer to this question is provided by certain obstetricians who have written about the longest of long-term developments in human childbearing.

9.2 Long-term developmental views of caesarean

The origins of the caesarean operation are often, and often erroneously, recounted in order to demonstrate its benefits (Dauphinee, 2004). Ancient myths and folk tales appear to hold some irresistible attraction for those advocating the benefits of caesarean. More recently, though, the history and prehistory of human birth have been attracting the attention not only of anthropologists (Kitzinger, 2000; Kay, 1982), but also of human palaeontologists (Rosenberg and Trevathan, 2002). In their attempts to justify the currently escalating caesarean rates and with variably successful results, medical practitioners have now also begun to jump on to the bandwagon of the prehistorical origins of human childbirth (Steer, 1998; Liston, 2003).

Obstetricians seem to derive considerable prestige from recounting the challenges encountered since time immemorial by the human female in giving birth physiologically. Steer is no exception and he attributes these challenges, and thus the increasing frequency of caesarean, to the human upright or bipedal posture and gait (1998). Because this posture and gait require a close alignment of the legs, they have supposedly had serious adverse implications for the woman's childbearing activities (1998:1052). This is due to the woman's pelvic canal having evolved to be relatively narrow (Tague and Lovejoy, 1986). The fetal head which needs to pass through the pelvis, however, is comparatively large due to the well-developed cerebral hemispheres.

Human palaeontologists, however, react to this line of thought by dismissing it as a mere 'popular perception' (Rosenberg and Trevathan, 2002:1199). They maintain that the challenges encountered during childbirth are not unique to the human woman. Comparisons are often made with our primate cousins, who may have more in common with our hominid antecedents than we, as human beings, do. Although the pelvic dimensions in the great apes are more generous, in the monkeys and lesser apes the ratio of fetal head size to pelvic capacity is similar to that of human beings. This means, for humans and lesser apes, that when the fetal head is in the mother's pelvis there is little if any unoccupied space. In fact, the bones of the fetal skull are likely to 'mould' in order to make better use of the limited space available. According to Rosenberg and Trevathan, the challenges of labour which face these smaller primates may also be similar to those facing the human woman.

On the basis of his slightly shaky palaeontology, Steer posits a competitive relationship between the fetus, who needs to be larger to improve her chance of survival, and the mother, who might prefer the baby to be smaller to ease the birth process. This allegedly competitive situation is said to contradict the assumption of human labour being 'harmonious . . . because it is natural' (Steer, 1998:1053). This feto-maternal competition, he argues, is still continuing to evolve. Perhaps predictably, Steer proposes caesarean as the solution to what he presents as an evolutionary predicament. While he argues that caesarean is a contribution to the on-going evolution of human beings, he does not need to state the role which obstetricians play in this process. We may at this point be forgiven for recalling the old chestnut of a joke:

Question What's the difference between God and an obstetrician?
Answer God doesn't think he's an obstetrician.

In support of his evolutionary argument, Steer quotes vast increases in the number of caesareans with no increase in perinatal mortality. In putting forward such a fallacious argument, he totally ignores the selection of women for a caesarean, compared with the absence of any selection for a vaginal birth. Further, there is no way of knowing how the perinatal and maternal mortality rates would have progressed had the 'caesarean epidemic' not broken out. The contribution of caesarean to human evolution is summarised by Steer's eager anticipation of this operation becoming the 'norm' (1998:1054), making vaginal birth effectively just a fall-back position. The spectre of 'prophylactic caesarean section' is clearly viewed as becoming a reality (Feldman and Freiman, 1985). In the event of Steer's prediction materialising, the fetal size would cease to be limited by the woman's pelvic dimensions. He anticipates, perhaps wistfully, that under such circumstances the woman would no longer even be *able* to give birth to her baby vaginally, because of the inevitable cephalo-pelvic disproportion (see Chapter 4). Thus Steer enthusiastically predicts that 'caesarean birth becomes necessary for the majority and is no longer just a choice' (1998:1054).

In further intended support of this doomsday scenario, Steer compares human women to dogs which have been seriously inbred, such as bulldogs. These poor creatures, courtesy of their human breeders, are often unable to give birth to their own offspring because of the excessive size of the puppy's head in relation to the mother dog's pelvis. The only woman who would not comply with this state of affairs is, according to Steer, the one who does not wish to protect her baby. If and when Steer's prediction comes to pass, though, it may be too late for anyone to take account of who needs to be protected.

Whether Steer's views of medical practitioners controlling the evolutionary process are common to his fellow professionals is not easy to assess. The fact that his views have not been widely lampooned and that the rise in the caesarean rate has not been checked may indicate that Steer may be accurately reflecting the views of his obstetrician colleagues (Kirby and Hanlon-Lundberg, 1999).

Another supporter for Steer's argument is also an obstetrician (Liston, 2003). He reaches a similar conclusion, though, by way of a marginally different route involving human ecology. In this case women are castigated, not for their pelvic size or large babies, but for their excess of both years and adipose tissue together with their lack of height. Surprisingly, Liston is at some pains to refute the 'widespread perception that the increasing caesarean rate is driven by obstetricians' (2003:561).

At the same time he deprecates women's inability to reach their maximum height potential, their tendency to become 'fat' and their delaying childbearing. In this way the cultural influences on women's behaviour and its effect on their bodies are linked to the caesarean decision.

These UK obstetricians' exceedingly long-term views of changes in the pattern of human childbearing are further illuminated by a North American study, which sought to identify whether caesarean shows a familial tendency (Varner et al, 1996). Clearly any such tendency would offer support to the evolutionary argument advanced by Steer. Varner and his colleagues, like so many of their medical brethren, appear convinced of the objectivity of medical diagnosis; this is manifested in their ability to see only the pathological condition, in this case 'dystocia' (see section 3.1.1). The cultural and other learned behaviour among the women in their sample would be more difficult for Varner and his colleagues to measure, so it is conveniently ignored. These researchers focus on this pathological uterine function, or dystocia, on intrauterine and childhood nutrition and on abnormalities of the bony pelvis. They quite correctly identify that young women who were born by caesarean are more likely to give birth by caesarean. What they neglect to address, though, is the reason for this intergenerational effect. The assumption is drawn that the causes of this effect are certainly purely physical, and probably genetic. Any social, cultural and learned influences, which are crucial to childbearing and which might either enhance or detract from the physical effects, do not feature. The evolutionary argument is supposedly supported by such medical research. It may be that such research serves only to further undermine a clearly shaky, and possibly flaky, line of reasoning.

Such a doomsday scenario, as is eagerly anticipated by medical writers, is viewed very differently by other health care professionals. In her analysis of American equivocation about 'woman initiated', 'planned pre-labour' caesareans, McCandlish contemplates the outcomes of such ambiguity (2006:206). Recognising that 'caesarean is not a benign intervention', she argues that acquiescing to maternal request is opening the door to the 'road to hell' (2006:206).

9.3 Medicalisation and women

The culture of childbearing appears to influence the incidence of caesarean, not only on an intergenerational basis, but also at a societal level (Cheung et al, 2005b). It may be that the various providers of maternity care are different in their influence on the consumers of care; this is likely to have repercussions on the acceptability of caesarean. Throughout this book, caesarean has emerged as both an example of and a result of the medicalisation of childbearing. While medicalisation may carry some benefits, its application to childbearing has been shown not to be free of disadvantages.

9.3.1 *The appeal of medicalisation*

The medical approach to childbirth may, of course, appeal to some childbearing women. In comparison to the midwife, the medical practitioner has the advantage that he is known to the woman. This may not necessarily involve personal acquaintance, but the woman is hardly likely to have reached childbearing age without having had some contact with medical practices. The same cannot be said for the midwife. It should not be surprising if the new mother-to-be is wary of meeting the midwife. The midwife is an unknown quantity. Unlike her medical colleagues, she rarely features in the popular media. It is perhaps for reasons like this that the childbearing woman may trust her medical practitioner and the birth choices which he recommends, rather than the midwife.

One aspect of medicalised care, which may attract the woman, is that she has some idea of what it looks like. She will have been in general practitioners' surgeries. She may have visited or spent time in hospital wards, or at least seen them on television. These environments are predictable, if not actually familiar, which may lead the woman to feel more secure with and more trusting of medical advice. Confidence in the personnel may lead the woman to be confident in the environment in which these practitioners practise, including the operating theatre.

By following a line of thought such as this, the woman is quite logically able to convince herself that a caesarean would not be such a bad birth choice, after all. This logical sequence is likely to appeal to the woman who is accustomed to a high standard of organisation and cleanliness in her mind, her body and her environment. It may be that this woman would not be comfortable with the adage, credited to Woody Allen and which originated in an only marginally different context, that if it's 'dirty', you must be 'doing it right'.

9.3.2 *Medicalisation and the woman's body*

The historical and prehistorical development of human birth has already been addressed (see section 9.2 above). So it is now appropriate to look forward to the implications of these developments for women and their bodies. As mentioned in Chapter 4, the spiralling caesarean rates in the Latin American countries and Brazil are now attracting more research attention (Belizán et al, 1999; Béhague et al, 2002a). The phenomenon identified by these groups of researchers may represent something other than just an inequitable system of health care which may be jeopardising the health, and even the lives, of childbearing women. The soaring caesarean rates in these countries may be an indication of a global trend for women who are obsessed with 'maintaining a sexually appealing body' (De Mello and

Souza, 1994). This obsession manifests itself, for example, in the prevalence of eating disorders in women. Another example of its appearance is found in the use of tobacco to curb the appetite in order to achieve the body shape which is considered desirable. As mentioned in Chapter 4, this body shape is not sought for the woman's gratification, but for the approval and enjoyment of her male sexual partner. In this way medicalisation, in the form of caesarean operations, is colluding with a male dominated society to achieve the oppression of women. As De Mello and Souza go on to observe, the woman's life and health is relegated to a very poor second place after the perceived necessity for a physically, that is sexually, attractive body.

In her presentation of a marginally different doomsday scenario from that painted by Steer, Bastian looks forward fearfully to the spread of the fashion for caesarean to the vast numbers of impoverished women in Latin America and Brazil (1999). The escalating trend towards caesarean as the norm is predicted to become a major public health problem. In such circumstances it is not the wealthy woman, as the originator of the caesarean fashion, who will be under threat; she will be able to pay for interventions to limit the danger. The real threat will be visited on the poverty-stricken families who have neither the knowledge nor the financial funds to call a halt to what will become a hazardous cycle of childbearing.

There are also other threats imposed by caesarean on women. Castro explores their nature in her disconcerting analysis (1999). She compares the unnecessary caesarean to other types of intervention, which may be perceived as forms of violence, which are inflicted on women during childbirth. The damage incurred by the caesarean is effectively interpreted as a violation of the woman's bodily integrity. This violence is aggravated by the woman's inability to give fully informed consent for the procedure. Such consent is clearly not possible when many of the long-term hazards are only now beginning to be recognised (please see section 7.1).

Castro's analysis of childbearing violence draws on one particularly apposite comparison. This is with the routine or prophylactic episiotomy which was practised throughout westernised maternity centres in the mid- to late twentieth century. This intervention was justified on the grounds of avoiding the risk of damage to the fetal brain and to the maternal tissues. Such damage would be aggravated by a long second stage and by the, allegedly, associated risks of fetal hypoxia. On the basis of these arguments, which clearly resonate with the current indications for caesarean (see section 5.2.2), performing and suturing episiotomies became a veritable growth industry. This late twentieth-century industry is comparable with the more recent 'caesarean epidemic'. It was not until a randomised controlled trial (Sleep et al, 1984) demonstrated the fallacy of the medical arguments for the use of episiotomy, that the routine practice began to be abandoned. A randomised controlled trial, though mooted, would hardly be likely to resolve the caesarean conundrum (Wax et al, 2004).

9.4 Risk

The comparison of caesarean with the late and unlamented routine episiotomy may be more relevant than is at first apparent. As mentioned already, a major aim of episiotomy was to reduce the risk of damage to the fetal cerebral structures. Secondarily, episiotomy was advocated for its ability to ensure that the vagina retained its prenatal muscle tone, in the supposed interests of sexual gratification. Similarly, caesarean has been criticised as an example of a fetocentric intervention (see section 5.5) which may also carry sexual benefits (7.1.4). The crucial difference is found, though, in the episiotomy having exposed the woman to risk for the benefit of her baby and her sexual partner. In the case of caesarean, on the other hand, the transfer of risk, though still to be borne by the woman on behalf of her baby and sexual partner, introduces risk being transferred from another source. The risk in the caesarean scenario has been shown by Wagner (2000) to be being transferred on to the woman from the medical practitioner. This transfer of risk opens a new meaning to the process of iatrogenesis, when the risk of harm visited on the woman is inflicted in order to avoid harm to the practitioner.

References

Aaronson, R.H. (1991) Grassroots strategies for promoting maternal and infant health. *Birth.* 18:2, 93–7.

Abitbol, M.M., Castillo, I., Taylor, U.B., Rochelson, B.L., Shmoys, S. and Monheit, A.G. (1993) Vaginal birth after cesarean section: the patient's point of view. *American Family Physician.* 47:1, 129–34.

ACOG (1999) Vaginal Birth After Previous Cesarean Delivery. American College of Obstetricians and Gynecologists, accessed July 2006, http://www.medem.com/search/article_display.cfm?path=n:&mstr=/ZZZ3CTZ6FIC.html&soc=ACOG&srch_typ=NAV_SERCH#top.

Adewuya, A.O., Ologun, Y.A. and Ibigbami, O.S. (2006) Post-traumatic stress disorder after childbirth in Nigerian women: prevalence and risk factors. *BJOG: An International Journal of Obstetrics and Gynaecology.* 113:3, 284–8.

AIMS/NCT (1997) A Charter for Ethical Research in Maternity Care. London: Association for Improvements in the Maternity Services and National Childbirth Trust.

Ainsworth, S. (2003) Back page. Cutting through time. *Practising Midwife.* 6:1, 42.

Akasheh, H.F. and Amarin, V. (2000) Caesarean sections at Queen Alia Military Hospital, Jordan: a six-year review. *Eastern Mediterranean Health Journal.* 6:1, 41–5.

Alfirevic, Z., Devane, D. and Gyte, G.M.L. (2006) Continuous cardiotocography (CTG) as a form of electronic fetal monitoring (EFM) for fetal assessment during labour. Cochrane Database of Systematic Reviews, Issue 3. Art. No.: CD006066. DOI: 10.1002/14651858.CD006066.

Al-Mufti, R.A., McCarthy, A. and Fisk, N.M. (1996) Obstetricians' personal choice and mode of delivery. *Lancet* 307, 544.

Al-Mufti, R.A., McCarthy, A. and Fisk, N.M. (1997) Survey of obstetricians' personal preference and discretionary practice. *European Journal of Obstetrics, Gynecology & Reproductive Biology.* 73:1, 1–4.

Alves, B. and Sheikh, A. (2005) Investigating the relationship between affluence and elective caesarean sections. *BJOG: An International Journal of Obstetrics and Gynaecology.* 112:7, 994–6.

Amu, O., Rajendran, S. and Bolaji, I.I. (1998) Should doctors perform an elective caesarean section on request? Maternal choice alone should not determine method of delivery. *British Medical Journal.* 317:7156, 463–5.

Anderson, T. (2006) Caesarean for non-medical reasons at term. *The Practising Midwife.* 9:1, 34–5.

Anim-Somuah, M., Smyth, R. and Howell, C. (2005) Epidural versus non-epidural or no analgesia in labour. Cochrane Database of Systematic Reviews, Issue 4. Art. No.: CD000331. DOI: 10.1002/14651858.CD000331.pub2.

Antonovsky, A. (1979) *Health, Stress and Coping*. San Francisco: Jossey-Bass.

ARM (2001) UK Midwifery Archives: Planning a good caesarean section. Caesareans under general anaesthetic. Association of Radical Midwives, accessed February 2006, http:// www.radmid.demon.co.uk/ csgood.htm#ga.

Arthur, D. and Payne, D. (2005) Maternal request for an elective caesarean section. *New Zealand College of Midwives Journal*. 33, 17–20.

Ayers, S. and Pickering, A.D. (2001) Do women get posttraumatic stress disorder as a result of childbirth? A prospective study of incidence. *Birth*. 28:2, 111–18.

Ayliffe, G.A.J. and English, M.P. (2003) *Hospital Infection: From Miasmas to MRSA*. Cambridge: Cambridge University Press.

Banks, M. (2000) *Home Birth Bound: Mending the Broken Weave*. Hamilton, New Zealand: Birthspirit.

Banks, M. (2001) Commentary on the Term Breech Trial. UK Midwifery Archives, accessed August 2006, http://www.radmid.demon.co.uk/breechbanks.htm.

Banks, M., Munro, J. and Spiby, H. (2001) But whose art frames the questions? *Practising Midwife*. 4:9, 34–6.

Barley, K., Aylin, P., Bottle, A. and Jarman, B. (2004) Social class and elective caesareans in the English NHS. *British Medical Journal*. 328:7453, 1399.

Barnabas, R.V., Carabin, H. and Garnett, G.P. (2002) The potential role of suppressive therapy for sex partners in the prevention of neonatal herpes: a health economic analysis. *Sexually Transmitted Infections*. 78:6, 425–9.

Barnard, A. (1999) Nursing and the primacy of technological progress. *International Journal of Nursing Studies*. 36:6, 435–42.

Barrett, J. (2005) Twin Birth Study: Study Protocol Maternal Infant and Reproductive Health Research Unit, Toronto, accessed April 2006, http://www.utoronto.ca/miru/index.htm.

Barrett, J.F.R. (2004) Delivery of the term twin. *Best Practice & Research in Clinical Obstetrics & Gynaecology*. 18:4, 625–30.

Barrett, G. and McCandlish, R. (2002) Caesarean section: better for your sex life? A review of the evidence. *MIDIRS Midwifery Digest*. 12:3, 377–9.

Barrett, G., Peacock, J., Victor, C.R. and Manyonda, I. (2005) Cesarean section and postnatal sexual health. *Birth*. 32:4, 306–11.

Basevi, V. and Lavender, T. (2000) Routine perineal shaving on admission in labour. Cochrane Database of Systematic Reviews, Issue 4. Art. No.: CD001236. DOI: 10.1002/ 14651858.CD001236.

Baskett, T.F. (1985) *Essential Management of Obstetric Emergencies*. Chichester: John Wiley.

Baskett, T.F. (2003) Emergency obstetric hysterectomy. *Journal of Obstetrics & Gynaecology*. 23:4, 353–5.

Bassett, K.L., Iyer, N. and Kazanjian, A. (2000) Defensive medicine during hospital obstetrical care: a byproduct of the technological age. *Social Science & Medicine*. 51:4, 523–37.

Bastian, H. (1999) Commentary: 'health has become secondary to a sexually attractive body'. *British Medical Journal*. 319:7222, 1402.

Baston, H. (2005) Midwifery basics: postnatal care. Post-operative care following caesarean. *Practising Midwife*. 8:2, 32–6.

Baxter, J. and MacFarlane, A. (2005) Postnatal caesarean care: evaluating the skill mix. *British Journal of Midwifery*. 13:6, 378–84.

Beckett, K. (2005) Choosing cesarean: feminism and the politics of childbirth in the United States. *Feminist Theory*. 6:3, 251–75.

Beech, B. (2000) Journalism and other influences. In Lee, B., Savage, W., Beech, B. and

Gillon, R., Too posh to push: the issue of caesarean section on demand. *RCM Midwives Journal*. 3(2): 52–3.

Beech, B.L. (1998/99) Book Review. *AIMS Journal*. 10:4, 21.

Beech, B. (2002a) Birthing a baby by the breech at home. *AIMS Journal*. 14:2, 4–5.

Beech, B.L. (2002b) What is Normal Birth? *AIMS Journal*. 13:4, 1–3.

Beech, B.L. (2003) Challenging the illusion of choice. *AIMS Journal*. 15:3, 1, 3–4.

Beech, B.L. (2003/04) Breech birth: a midwifery approach. *AIMS Journal*. 15:4, 5–6.

Beech, B.L. (2004) NICE guidelines for caesarean section. *AIMS Journal*. 16:2, 1–3.

Béhague, D.P., Victora, C.G. and Barros, F.C. (2002) Consumer demand for caesarean sections in Brazil: population based birth cohort study linking ethnographic and epidemiological methods. *British Medical Journal*. 324:7343, 942–5.

Belizán, J.M., Althabe, F., Barros, F.C. and Alexander, S. (1999) Rates and implications of caesarean sections in Latin America: ecological study. *British Medical Journal*. 319:7222, 1397–400.

Benatar, S.R. (2004) Health Challenges: South Africa and the World Centenary Lecture, Rhodes University, accessed February 2006, www.ru.ac.za/centenary/lectures/Rhodes_Univ_Health_Challenges.pdf.

Berryman, J.C. and Windridge, K.C. (1995) *Motherhood after 35*. Leicester: University of Leicester.

Bettcher, D. and Lee, K. (2002) Globalisation and public health. *Journal of Epidemiology and Community Health*. 56:1, 8–17.

Bewley, S. and Cockburn. J. (2004) Should doctors perform caesarean for 'Informed choice' alone? In Kirkham, M. (ed.), *Informed Choice in Maternity Care*. Basingstoke: Palgrave Macmillan, ch. 9, pp. 185–210.

Biggar, R.J., Miotti, P.G., Taha, T.E., Mtimavalye, L., Broadhead R., Justesen, A., Yellin, F., Liomba, G., Miley, W., Waters, D., Chiphangwi, J.D. and Goedert, J.J. (1996) Perinatal intervention trial in Africa: effect of a birth canal cleansing intervention to prevent HIV transmission. *Lancet*. 347:9016, 1647–50.

BIRTHCHOICE (2006) Scottish Maternity Statistics, accessed 6 February 2006, http://www.birthchoiceuk.com/Frame.htm.

Bjorklund, K. (2002) Minimally invasive surgery for obstructed labour: a review of symphysiotomy during the twentieth century (including 5000 cases). *BJOG: An International Journal of Obstetrics and Gynaecology*. 109:3, 225–6.

Black, C., Kaye, J.A. and Jick, H. (2005) Cesarean delivery in the United Kingdom: time trends in the General Practice Research Database. *Obstetrics and Gynecology*. 106:1, 151–5.

Blanchette, H.A., Nayak, S. and Erasmus, S. (1999) Comparison of the safety and efficacy of intravaginal misoprostol (prostaglandin E1) with those of dinoprostone (prostaglandin E2) for cervical ripening and induction of labor in a community hospital. *American Journal of Obstetrics and Gynecology*. 180:6 Pt 1, 1551–9.

Blumenfeld-Kosinski, R. (1990) *Not of Woman Born: Representations of Caesarean Birth in Medieval and Renaissance Culture*. Ithaca and London: Cornell University Press.

Boenigk, M. (2006) Last word: time to get out of bed. *The Practising Midwife*. 9:5, 62.

Bolbos, G. and Sindos, M. (2005) The Bolbos technique for the management of uncontrollable intra-caesarean uterine bleeding. *Archives of Gynecology and Obstetrics*. 272:2, 142–4.

Bonica, J.J. (1990) History of pain concepts and therapies. In Bonica, J.J. (ed.), *The Management of Pain* (2nd edn). Philadelphia: Lea & Febiger.

Bost, B.W. (2003) Cesarean delivery on demand: what will it cost? *American Journal of Obstetrics and Gynecology*. 188:6, 1418–21.

Botting, B. (1995) *The health of our children. Decennial supplement.* London: HMSO Office of Population Censuses and Surveys, p. 71.

Boyd, S. (2003) Coffin Birth, accessed November 2005, http://www.livejournal.com/community/rigormortis/29114.html.

Brady, M., Kinn, S. and Stuart, P. (2003) Preoperative fasting for adults to prevent perioperative complications. Cochrane Database of Systematic Reviews, Issue 4. Art. No.: CD004423. DOI: 10.1002/14651858.CD004423.

Broach, J. and Newton, N. (1988) Food and beverages in labour. Part II: the effects of cessation of oral intake during labour. *Birth.* 15, 88–92.

Brunner, L.S. and Suddarth, D.S. (1992) The Textbook of Adult Nursing. London: Chapman & Hall.

Buckley, S.J. (2004) Labour and birth: what disturbs birth? *MIDIRS Midwifery Digest.* 14:3, 353–9.

Buekens, P., Curtis, S. and Alayon, S. (2003) Demographic and health surveys: caesarean section rates in sub-Saharan Africa. *British Medical Journal.* 326:7381, 136.

Bujold, E., Bujold, C., Hamilton, E.F., Harel, F. and Gauthier, R.J. (2002) The impact of a single-layer or double-layer closure on uterine rupture. *American Journal of Obstetrics and Gynecology.* 186:6, 1326–30.

Burrows, J. (2001) The parturient woman: can there be room for more than 'one person with full and equal rights inside a single human skin'? *Journal of Advanced Nursing.* 33:5, 689–95.

Cahill, H. (1999) An Orwellian scenario: court ordered caesarean section and women's autonomy. *Nursing Ethics.* Nov. 6:6, 494–505.

Calvert, I. and Stinson, C. (In press) *Caesarian Wound Surveillance.*

Carroll, L. (2000) *Alice's Adventures in Wonderland and Through the Looking Glass.* London: Signet Classic.

Casetti, E. (2003) Power shifts and economic development: when will China Overtake the USA? *Journal of Peace Research.* 40:6, 661–75.

Castro, A. (1999) Commentary: increase in caesarean sections may reflect medical control not women's choice, commentary on Belizán, J.M., Althabe, F., Barros, F.C. and Alexander, S. (1999) Rates and implications of caesarean sections in Latin America: ecological study. *British Medical Journal.* 319:1397–1400, pp. 1401–2.

Caufield, H. (1999) A review of the law on enforced caesareans. *MIDIRS Midwifery Digest.* 9:1 117–19.

Cesario, S.K. (2004) Reevaluation of Friedman's Labor Curve: a pilot study. *JOGNN: Journal of Obstetric, Gynecologic and Neonatal Nursing.* 33:6, 713–22.

Chalmers, B. (2004) Globalisation and perinatal health care. *BJOG: An International Journal of Obstetrics and Gynaecology.* 111:9, 889–91.

Chama, C.M., Wanonyi, I.K. and Usman, J.D. (2004) From low-lying implantation to placenta praevia: a longitudinal ultrasonic assessment. *Journal of Obstetrics & Gynaecology.* 24: 5, 516–8.

Chamberlain, G., Wraight, A. and Crowley, P. (eds) (1997) Home Births: The Report of the 1994 Confidential Enquiry by the National Birthday Trust Fund.

Cheung, N.F. (2000) The childbearing experiences of Chinese and Scottish women in Scotland, unpublished PhD Thesis. University of Edinburgh.

Cheung, N.F. (2006) Personal communication.

Cheung, N.F., Mander, R. and Cheng, L. (2005a) The 'doula-midwives' in Shanghai. *Evidence-Based Midwifery.* 3:2, 73–9.

Cheung, N.F., Mander, R., Cheng, L., Yang, X.Q. and Chen, V.Y. (2005b) 'Informed choice' in the context of caesarean decision-making in China. *Evidence-Based Midwifery*. 3:1, 33–8.

Cheung, N.F., Mander, R., Cheng, L., Chen, V.Y., Yang, X.Q., Qian, H.P. and Qian, J.Y. (2006) 'Zuoyuezi' after caesarean in China: an interview survey. *International Journal of Nursing Studies*. 43:2, 193–202.

Cheyne, H., Dunlop, A., Shields, N. and Mathers, A.M. (2003) A randomised controlled trial of admission electronic fetal monitoring in normal labour. *Midwifery*. 19:3, 221–9.

Churchill, H. (2003) *Caesarean Birth: Experience, Practice and History*. Hale: Books for Midwives.

Churchill, H., Savage, W. and Francome, C. (2006) *Caesarean Birth in Britain*. London: Middlesex University Press.

Clement, S. (1995) *The Caesarean Experience*. London: Pandora.

Clement, S. (2001) The Caesarean Experience, Chapter 9 in Drife, J. and Walker, J. (eds), *Best Practice and Research in Clinical Obstetrics and Gynaecology*. 15:1, 165–78.

Cochrane, A.L. (1972) *Effectiveness and Efficiency: Random Reflections on Health Services*. London: Nuffield Provincial Hospitals Trust.

Cochrane Library (2005) The Cochrane Collaboration. John Wiley & Sons Ltd, accessed December 2005, http://www.mrw.interscience.wiley.com/cochrane/cochrane_search_fs.html.

Cohain, J.S. and Yoselis, A. (2004) Caesareans and low-risk women in Israel. *Practising Midwife*. 7:7, 28–31.

Cohen, D. (2005) My six day experience in the Middle East. *British Medical Journal*. 330:7489, 474–7.

Comer, M.W. (1921) What are the principal complications of pregnancy? *The British Journal of Nursing*. November 19, p. 314, accessed January 2006, rcnarchive.rcn.org.uk/data /VOLUME067-1921/page314–volume67–19th November1921.pdf – Supplemental Result.

Cooper, G.M. and McClure, J.H. (2004) Anaesthesia. Chapter 9 in Lewis, G. (2004) *Why Mothers Die 2000–2002 – Report on confidential enquiries into maternal deaths in the United Kingdom*. London: CEMACH, RCOG.

Coyle, M.E., Smith, C.A. and Peat, B. (2005) Cephalic version by moxibustion for breech presentation. Cochrane Database of Systematic Reviews, Issue 2. Art. No.: CD003928. DOI: 10.1002/14651858.CD003928.pub2.

Coyle, P. (1992) General Anaesthesia for caesarean section. Update in *Anaesthesia*. 2:4, 1–2, accessed February 2006, http://www.nda.ox.ac.uk/wfsa/html/u02/u02_006.htm.

Craigin, E.B. (1916) Conservatism in obstetrics. *New York Medical Journal*. 104, 1–3.

Crawford, J.S. (1986) Maternal mortality from Mendelson's syndrome. *The Lancet*. 1, 920–1.

Cronk, M. (2005) Hands off that breech! *AIMS Journal*. 17:1, 1, 3–4.

Dathe, O., Lutz-Friedrich, R., Grubert, T., Knobbe, A. and Kästner, R. (1998) Postoperative complications following 201 gynecological and obstetrical surgical interventions in HIV-infected women. 12th World AIDS Conference, Geneva (abstract #13391).

Dauphinee, J.D. (2004) VBAC: safety for the patient and the nurse. *Journal of Obstetric, Gynecologic and Neonatal Nursing*. 33:1, 105–15.

De Costa, C.M. (2001) 'Ript from the womb': a short history of caesarean section. *Medical Journal of Australia*. 174:1, 97–100.

De Mello, E. and Souza, C. (1994) C-sections as ideal births: The cultural constructions of beneficence and patients' rights in Brazil. *Cambridge Quarterly Healthcare Ethics*. 3, 358–66.

De Vries, R.G. (1993) A cross-national view of the status of midwives. In Riska, E. and Wegar, K. (eds), *Gender Work and Medicine: Women and the Medical Division of Labour*. London: Sage, Ch. 6, pp. 131–46.

Declercq, E. and Viisainen, K. (2001) Appendix: The politics of numbers. In Abram, S., De Vries, R., Marland, H., Van Teijlingen, E. and Wrede, S. (eds), *Birth by Design: Pregnancy, Maternity Care and Midwifery in North America and Europe*. London: Routledge, p. 267.

Den Exter, A., Hermans, H., Doslajak, M. and Busse, R. (2004) *Health Care Systems in Transition, the Netherlands*. Copenhagen, Denmark: European Observatory on Health Care Systems.

Dennis, B. (1994) Care study: severe needle phobia. *Midwives Chronicle*. 107:1273, 58–61.

Derrick, D.C. (2005) Term breech trial follow up. *AIMS Journal*. 17:2, 9.

Dessole, S., Cosmi, E., Balata, A., Uras, L., Caserta, D., Capobianco, G. and Ambrosini, G. (2004) Accidental fetal lacerations during cesarean delivery: experience in an Italian level III university hospital. *American Journal of Obstetrics and Gynecology*. 191:5, 1673–7.

Devane, D. and Lalor, J. (2005) Midwives' visual interpretation of intrapartum cardiotocographs: intra- and inter-observer agreement. *Journal of Advanced Nursing*. 52:2, 133–41.

DHSS (1970) Standing Maternity and Midwifery Advisory Committee, Domiciliary midwifery and maternity bed needs: report of a sub-committee. Peel Report. London: HMSO.

Di Renzo, G.C. (2003) Tocophobia: a new indication for cesarean delivery? *Journal of Maternal-Fetal and Neonatal Medicine*. 13:4, 217.

Dick-Read, G. (1933) *Natural Childbirth*. London: W. Heinemann.

Dickson, M.J. and Willett, M. (1999) Midwives would prefer a vaginal delivery. *British Medical Journal*. 319: 7215, 1008.

DiMatteo, M.R., Morton, S.C., Lepper, H.S., Damush, T.M., Carney, M.F., Pearson, M. and Kahn, K.L. (1996) Cesarean childbirth and psychosocial outcomes: a meta-analysis. *Health Psychology*. 15:4, 303–14.

Dodd, J. and Crowther, C. (2004a) Vaginal birth after Caesarean versus elective repeat Caesarean for women with a single prior Caesarean birth: a systematic review of the literature. *Australian and New Zealand Journal of Obstetrics and Gynaecology*. 44:5, 387–91.

Dodd, J.M. and Crowther, C.A. (2004b) Elective repeat caesarean section versus induction of labour for women with a previous caesarean birth. (Protocol) Cochrane Database of Systematic Reviews, Issue 3. Art. No.: CD004906. DOI: 10.1002/14651858.CD004906.

Dodd, J.M. and Crowther, C.A. (2005) Evidence-based care of women with a multiple pregnancy. *Best Practice and Research in Clinical Obstetrics and Gynaecology*. 19:1, 131–53.

Dodd, J., Crowther, C.A. and Huertas, E. (2003) Planned elective repeat caesarean section versus planned vaginal birth for women with a previous caesarean birth (Protocol for a Cochrane Review). In Cochrane Library, Issue 3, Oxford: Update Software.

Dodd, J.M., Crowther, C.A., Huertas, E., Guise, J.M. and Horey, D. (2004) Planned elective repeat caesarean section versus planned vaginal birth for women with a previous caesarean birth. Cochrane Database of Systematic Reviews, Issue 4. Art. No.: CD004224. DOI: 10.1002/14651858.CD004224.pub2.

DoH (1993) *Changing Childbirth*. Report of the Expert Maternity Group. Practice. Department of Health: HMSO.

DoH (2004) Maternity Statistics England 2002-03, accessed February 2006, www.dh.gov.uk/assetRoot/04/08/08/23/04080823.pdf.

DoH (2005a) Action on health care associated infections in England: Summary of responses to the consultation, accessed February 2006, http://www.dh.gov.uk/Consultations/ResponsesToConsultations/ResponsesToConsultationsDocumentSummary/fs/en?CONTENT_ID=4123671andchk=uxz/Z7.

DoH (2005b) Maternity statistics England 2003-04, accessed March 2006, http://www.dh.gov.uk/PublicationsAndStatistics/Publications/PublicationsStatistics/PublicationsStatisticsArticle/fs/en?CONTENT_ID=4107060andchk=IY7Bqa.

DoH (2006) MRSA surveillance system results. Department of Health, London, accessed May 2006, http://www.dh.gov.uk/PublicationsAndStatistics/Publications/PublicationsStatistics/PublicationsStatisticsArticle/fs/en?CONTENT_ID=4085951andchk=HBt2QD.

Doherty, J.P., Norton, E.C. and Veney, J.E. (2001) China's one-child policy: the economic choices and consequences faced by pregnant women. *Social Science and Medicine*. 52:5, 745–61.

Downe, S. (2004) *Normal Childbirth: Evidence and Debate*. Edinburgh: Churchill Livingstone.

Downie, L. (2006) Elective caesarean section: the baby's experience. *Birth and Beyond* 26:14, accessed July 2006, http://www.birthresourcecentre.org.uk/BandBdownload.htm.

Doyal, L. (2001) Education and debate. Sex, gender, and health: the need for a new approach. *British Medical Journal*. 323:7320, 1061–3.

Drayton, S. (1990) Midwifery Care in the First Stage of Labour. In Alexander, J., Levy, V. and Roch, S. (eds), *Intrapartum Care: A Research-Based Approach*. London: Macmillan, pp. 24–41.

Dresner, M.R. and Freeman, J.M. (2001) Anaesthesia for caesarean section, Chapter 8 in Drife, J. and Walker, J. (eds), *Clinical Obstetrics and Gynaecology*. 15:1, 127–44.

Drife, J. (2004) Other direct deaths. In Lewis, G. (ed.), Why Mothers Die 2000–2002 – Report on confidential enquiries into maternal deaths in the United Kingdom. London: CEMACH, RCOG, p. 118.

ECS (2005) European Collaborative Study. Mother to child transmission of HIV infection in the era of highly active antiretroviral therapy. *Clinical Infectious Diseases* 40:458–65.

Edwards, N. (2003) The choice is yours – or is it? *AIMS Journal*. 15:3, 9–12.

Edwards, N. (2005) *Birthing Autonomy: Women's Experiences of Planning Home Births*. Abingdon: Routledge.

EGAMS (2003) *Expert Group on Acute Maternity Services*. Edinburgh: Scottish Executive.

Enkin, M. (1992) Can changes in practice be implemented? In Chard, T. and Richards, M.P.M. (eds), *Obstetrics in the 1990s: Current Controversies*. London: Mac Keith Press, pp. 212–19.

Enkin, M., Keirse, M.J.N.C. and Chalmers, I. (1995) A Guide to Effective Care in Pregnancy and Childbirth (2nd edn). Oxford: Oxford University Press.

Entwistle, D.R. and Alexander, K.L. (1987) Long-term effects of cesarean delivery on parents' beliefs and children's schooling. *Developmental Psychology*. 23:5, 676–82.

Eriksson, C., Jansson, L. and Hamberg, K. (2006) Women's experiences of intense fear related to childbirth investigated in a Swedish qualitative study. *Midwifery*. 22:3, 240–8.

Ettinger, F. (2001) Turn the bag around . . . nurses seem so used to dealing with urine they forget it might embarrass the patients to have theirs displayed. *Nursing Standard*. 15:34, 26.

EWTD (2003) Council of the European Union. 2003. Directive 2003/88/EC of the European

Parliament and the Council of 4 November 2003 concerning certain aspects of the organisation of working time (accessed July 2006).

Farah, N., Geary, M., Connolly, G. and McKenna, P. (2003) The caesarean section rate in the Republic of Ireland in 1998. *Irish Medical Journal*. 96:8, 242–3.

Faundes, A., Guarisi, T. and Pinto-Neto, A.M. (2001) The risk of urinary incontinence of parous women who delivered only by cesarean section. *International Journal of Gynaecology and Obstetrics*. 72:1, 41–6.

Fawcett, J., Tulman, L. and Spedden, J.P. (1994) Responses to vaginal birth after cesarean section. *JOGNN: Journal of Obstetric, Gynecologic and Neonatal Nursing*. 23:3, 253–9.

Feldman, G.B. and Freiman, J.A. (1985) Prophylactic cesarean section at term? *New England Journal of Medicine*. 312:19, 1264–7.

Filc, D. (2005) The health business under neo-liberalism: the Israeli case. *Critical Social Policy*. 25:2, 180–97.

Flamm, B.L. (2001a) Vaginal birth after caesarean (VBAC). *Best Practice and Research in Clinical Obstetrics and Gynaecology*. 15:1, 81–92.

Flamm. B.L. (2001b) In the literature. Vaginal birth after cesarean and the New England Journal of Medicine: a strange controversy. *Birth*. 28:4, 276–9.

Fleming, V. (2000) The midwifery partnership in New Zealand: past history or a new way forward. In Kirkham, M. (ed.), *The Midwife-Mother Relationship*. London: Macmillan, p. 193.

Fok, W.Y., Chan, L.W., Leung, T.Y. and Lau, T.K. (2005) Maternal experience of pain during external cephalic version at term. *Acta Obstetricia et Gynecologica Scandinavica*. 84:8, 748–51.

Francome, C., Savage, W., Churchill, H. and Lewison, H. (1993) Caesarean Birth in Britain. London: Middlesex University Press in association with The National Childbirth Trust.

Frei, I.A. (2005) Personal communication.

Friedman, E.A. (1954) Graphic analysis of labor. *American Journal of Obstetrics and Gynecology*. 68, 1568–75.

Frost, L., Pederson, M. and Seiersen, E. (1989) Changes in hygienic procedures reduce infection following Caesarean section. *Journal of Hospital Infection*. 13, 143–8.

Funk, S.G., Champagne, M.T., Wiese, R.A. and Tornquist, E.M. (1991) Barriers: the barriers to research utilization scale. *Applied Nursing Research*. 4:1, 39–45.

Ganong W.F. (1997) *Review of Medical Physiology*, 18th edn. Stamford, CO: Appleton & Lange.

Garforth, S. and Garcia, J. (1987) Admitting – a weakness or a strength? Routine admission of a woman in labour . . . current English midwifery practice. *Midwifery*. 3:1, 10–24.

Garrey, M.M., Govan, A.D.T., Hodge, C.H. and Callander, R. (1969) *Obstetrics Illustrated*. Edinburgh: Churchill Livingstone.

Gates, S., Brocklehurst, P. and Davis, L.J. (2002) Prophylaxis for venous thromboembolic disease in pregnancy and the early postnatal period. Cochrane Database of Systematic Reviews, Issue 2. Art. No.: CD001689. DOI: 10.1002/14651858.CD001689.

Gerber, A.H. (1974) Accidental incision of the fetus during cesarean delivery. *International Journal of Obstetrics and Gynecology*. 12, 46–8.

Gielchinsky, Y., Rojansky, N., Fasouliotis, S.J. and Ezra, Y. (2002) Placenta accreta – summary of 10 years: a survey of 310 cases. *Placenta*. 23:2–3, 210–14.

Glantz, J.C. and McNanley, T.J. (1997) Active management of labor: a meta-analysis of Cesarean delivery rates for dystocia in nulliparas. *Obstetrical and Gynecological Survey*. 52:8, 497–505.

Glazener, C.M., Herbison, G.P., Macarthur, C., Grant, A. and Wilson, P.D. (2005)

Randomised controlled trial of conservative management of postnatal urinary and faecal incontinence: six year follow up. *British Medical Journal*. 330:7487, 337.

Glezerman, M. (2006) Five years to the term breech trial: the rise and fall of a randomized controlled trial. *American Journal of Obstetrics and Gynecology*. 194:1, 20–5.

Gocmen, A., Gocmen, M. and Saraoglu, M. (2002) Early post-operative feeding after caesarean delivery. *Journal of International Medical Research*. 30:5, 506–11.

Godden, D. (2005) Providing health services to rural and remote communities. *Journal of Royal College of Physicians Edinburgh*. 35, 294–5.

Goer, H.A. (2004) Consumer viewpoint. Humanizing birth: a global grassroots movement. *Birth*. 31:4, 308–14.

Goldberg, R.P., Abramov, Y., Botros, S., Miller, J.J., Gandhi, S., Nickolov, A., Sherman, W. and Sand, P.K. (2005) Delivery mode is a major environmental determinant of stress urinary incontinence: results of the Evanston-Northwestern Twin Sisters Study. *American Journal of Obstetrics and Gynecology*. 193:6, 2149–53.

Goldstick, O., Weissman, A. and Drugan, A. (2003) The circadian rhythm of 'urgent' operative deliveries. *Israel Medical Association Journal*. 5:8, 564–6.

Gorer, G. (1965) *Death, Grief and Mourning in Contemporary Britain*. London: Cresset Press.

Gould, D. (2000) Normal labour: a concept analysis. *Journal of Advanced Nursing*. 31:2, 418–27.

Graham, I.D. (1997) *Episiotomy: Challenging Obstetric Interventions*. Oxford: Blackwell Science.

Graham, W.J., Hundley, V., McCheyne, A.L., Hall, M.H., Gurney, E. and Milne, J. (1999) An investigation of women's involvement in the decision to deliver by caesarean section. *British Journal of Obstetrics and Gynaecology*. 106:3, 213–20.

Green, B. (2005) Midwives' coping methods for managing birth uncertainties. *British Journal of Midwifery*. 13:5, 293–8.

Green, J.M. and Baston, H.A. (2003) Feeling in control during labor: concepts, correlates, and consequences. *Birth*. 30:4, 235–47.

Gregory, K.D., Korst, L.M., Cane, P., Platt, L.D. and Kahn, K. (1999) Vaginal birth after cesarean and uterine rupture rates in California. *Obstetrics and Gynecology*. 94:6, 985–9.

Groeschel, N. and Glover, P. (2001)The partograph used daily but rarely questioned. *Australian Journal of Midwifery*. 14:3, 22–7.

Guise, J.M., McDonagh, M.S., Osterweil, P., Nygren, P., Chan, B.K. and Helfand, M. (2004) Systematic review of the incidence and consequences of uterine rupture in women with previous caesarean section. *British Medical Journal*. 329:7456, 19–25.

Hall, M.H. (2004) Haemorrhage. In Lewis, G. (ed.), Why Mothers Die 2000–2002 – Report on confidential enquiries into maternal deaths in the United Kingdom. London: CEMACH, RCOG, p. 86.

Hannah, M., Hannah, W., Hewson, S., Hodnett, E., Saigal, S. and Willan, A. (2000) Planned caesarean section versus planned vaginal birth for breech presentation at term: a randomised multicentre trial. Breech Trial Collaborative Group. *Lancet*. 356, 1375–83.

Hannah, M.E., Whyte, H., Hannah, W.J., Hewson, S., Amankwah, K., Cheng, M., Gafni, A., Guselle, P., Helewa, M., Hodnett, E.D., Hutton, E., Kung, R., McKay, D., Ross, S., Saigal, S. and Willan, A. (2004) Term Breech Trial Collaborative Group. Maternal outcomes at 2 years after planned cesarean section versus planned vaginal birth for breech presentation at term: the international randomized Term Breech Trial. *American Journal of Obstetrics and Gynecology*. 191:3, 917–27.

Harer, W.B. (2002) Vaginal birth after cesarean delivery: current status. *JAMA: Journal of the American Medical Association.* 287:20, 2627–30.

Harper, A. (2004) Genital tract sepsis. In Lewis, G. (ed.), Why Mothers Die 2000–2002 – Report on confidential enquiries into maternal deaths in the United Kingdom. London: CEMACH, RCOG, p. 109.

Harris, L.H. (2001) Counselling women about choice. In Drife, J. and Walker J. (eds), *Best Practice and Research in Clinical Obstetrics and Gynaecology.* 15:1, 93–107.

Hedberg, B. and Larsson, U.S. (2004) Environmental elements affecting the decision-making process in nursing practice. *Journal of Clinical Nursing.* 13:3, 316–24.

Helen (2004) How soon ttc after section? Accessed November 2005, http://www.babyworld.co.uk/wb/default.asp?action=91andread=20424andfid=45andprv=17065andnxt=17404.

Helmy, W.H., Jolaoso, A.S., Ifaturoti, O.O., Afify, S.A. and Jones, M.H. (2002) The decision-to-delivery interval for emergency caesarean section: is 30 minutes a realistic target? *BJOG: An International Journal of Obstetrics and Gynaecology.* 109:5, 505–8.

Hem, E. and Børdahl, P.E. (2003) Max Sanger – father of the modern caesarean section. *Gynecologic and Obstetric Investigation.* 55:3, 127–9.

Hemminki, E. (1986) Effects of cesarean section on fertility and abortions. *Journal of Reproductive Medicine.* 31:7 620–4.

Hemminki, E. (1996) Impact of caesarean section on future pregnancy: a review of cohort studies. *Paediatric and Perinatal Epidemiology.* 10:4, 366–79.

Hemminki, E. and Merilainen, J. (1996) Long-term effects of cesarean sections: ectopic pregnancies and placental problems. *American Journal of Obstetrics and Gynecology.* 174:5, 1569–74.

Hemminki, E., Graubard, B.I., Hoffman, H.J., Mosher, W.D. and Fetterly, K. (1985) Cesarean section and subsequent fertility: results from the 1982 National Survey of Family Growth. *Fertility and Sterility.* 43:4, 520–8.

Herbert, W. (2003) Fetal lacerations at elective/non emergency caesarean sections. NHS Litigation Authority Review NHSLA, 28, 8–9.

Hewson, B. (1994) Court-ordered caesarean: ethical triumph or surgical rape? *AIMS Journal.* 6:2, 1–5.

Hicks, C. (2004) Midwifery research: some ethical considerations. In Frith, L. and Draper, H. (eds), *Ethics and Midwifery* (2nd edn). Edinburgh: Books for Midwives.

Hicks, T.L., Goodall, S.F., Quattrone, E.M. and Lydon-Rochelle, M.T. (2004) Postpartum sexual functioning and method of delivery: summary of the evidence. *Journal of Midwifery and Women's Health.* 49:5, 430–6.

Hillan, E. (1991a) Caesarean section: maternal risks . . . part 1. *Nursing Standard.* 5:48, 26–9.

Hillan, E. (1991b) Caesarean section: perinatal risks . . . part 2. *Nursing Standard.* 5:49, 37–9.

Hillan, E.M. (1992a) Short-term morbidity associated with caesarean section. *Journal of Clinical Nursing.* 1:2, 107–8.

Hillan, E.M. (1992b) Maternal–infant attachment following caesarean delivery. *Journal of Clinical Nursing.* 1:1, 33–7.

Hillan, E.M. (1992c) Short-term morbidity associated with cesarean delivery. *Birth.* 19:4, 190–4.

Hillan, E.M. (1995) Postoperative morbidity following Caesarean delivery. *Journal of Advanced Nursing.* 22:6, 1035–42.

Hillan, E. (2000) The aftermath of caesarean delivery. *MIDIRS Midwifery Digest.* 10:1, 70–2.

Hinchliff, S.M. and Montague, S.E. (1988) *Physiology for Nursing Practice.* London: Baillière Tindall.

HMSO (1996) *Report on Confidential Enquiries into Maternal Deaths in the UK 1991–93.* London: HMSO.

HoC (1992) Health Committee Second Report, Maternity Services, Chair: N. Winterton. London: HMSO House of Commons.

Hodnett, E.D., Gates, S., Hofmeyr, G.J. and Sakala, C. (2003) Continuous support for women during childbirth. Cochrane Database of Systematic Reviews, Issue 3. Art. No.: CD003766. DOI: 10.1002/14651858.CD003766.

Hofberg, K. and Brockington, I. (2000) Tokophobia: An unreasoning dread of childbirth. A series of 26 cases. *British Journal of Psychiatry.* 176, 83–5.

Hofmann, B. (2002) Technological medicine and the autonomy of man. *Medicine, Health Care and Philosophy.* 5, 2157–67.

Hofmeyr, G.J. and Gyte, G. (2004) Interventions to help external cephalic version for breech presentation at term. Cochrane Database of Systematic Reviews, Issue 1. Art. No.: CD000184. DOI: 10.1002/14651858.CD000184.pub2.

Hofmeyr, G.J. and Hannah, M.E. (2003) Planned caesarean section for term breech delivery. Cochrane Database of Systematic Reviews, Issue 2. Art. No.: CD000166. DOI: 10.1002/14651858.CD000166.

Hofmeyr, G.J. and Kulier, R. (2000) Cephalic version by postural management for breech presentation. Cochrane Database of Systematic Reviews, Issue 3. Art. No.: CD000051. DOI: 10.1002/14651858.CD000051.

Homer, C.S.E., Davis, G.K., Cooke, M. and Barclay, L.M. (2002) Women's experiences of continuity of midwifery care in a randomised controlled trial in Australia. *Midwifery.* 18:2, 102–12.

Hook, B., Kiwi, R., Amini, S.B., Fanaroff, A. and Hack, M. (1997) Neonatal morbidity after elective repeat cesarean section and trial of labor. *Pediatrics.* 100:3, Pt 1, 348–53.

Höpker, M., Fleckenstein, G., Heyl, W., Sattler, B. and Emons, G. (2002) Placenta percreta in week 10 of pregnancy with consecutive hysterectomy: case report. *Human Reproduction.* 17:3, 817–20.

Horey, D., Weaver, J. and Russell, H. (2004) Information for pregnant women about caesarean birth. Cochrane Database of Systematic Reviews Issue 1. Art. No.: CD003858. DOI: 10.1002/14651858.CD003858.pub2.

Hunt, J. (1801) Historical surgery, or the progress of the science of medicine: on inflammation, mortification, and gun-shot wounds. Loughborough [s.n.].

Hutton, E.K. and Hofmeyr, G.J. (2006) External cephalic version for breech presentation before term. Cochrane Database of Systematic Reviews 2006, Issue 1. Art. No.: CD000084. DOI: 10.1002/14651858.CD000084.pub2.

Hyder, A.A. and Morrow, R.H. (2001) Disease burden: measurement and trends. In Merson, M.H., Black, R.E. and Mills, A.J. (eds), *International Public Health: Diseases, Programs, Systems, and Policies.* Gaithersburg, MD: Aspen, pp. 1–51.

ICAN (2004) Local groups found to raise awareness of caesarean, accessed July 2006, http://www.ican-online.org/.

ICAN (2006) International Cesarean Awareness Network Inc, accessed July 2006, http://www.ican-online.org/.

ICM (2005) Definition of a Midwife, International Confederation of Midwives Council meeting, 19th July, Brisbane, Australia.

Iglesias, S., Burn, R. and Saunders, L.D. (1991) Reducing the cesarean section rate in a rural community hospital. *CMAJ Canadian Medical Association Journal.* 145:11, 1459–64.

Illich, I. (1976) *Limits to Medicine: Medical Nemesis: The Expropriation of Health*. London: Boyars.

Illich, I. (1995) Death undefeated from medicine to medicalisation to systematisation. *British Medical Journal*. 311, 1652–3.

IMA (2005) IMA Statistics, Independent Midwives Association, accessed July 2006, http://www.independentmidwives.org.uk/.

Inch, S. (1986) When the midwife misses out. *Nursing Times*. 82:22, 67.

ISD (2004) Live births by mode and hospital, accessed December 2006, http://www. isdscotland.org/isd/files/mat_bb_table5.xls.

ISD (2005a) Childhood mortality number of deaths by age, accessed March 2006, http://www.isdscotland.org/isd/info3.jsp?pContentID=2511andp_applic=CCC&p_service=Content.show&.

ISD (2005b) Live births by mode and hospital, accessed March 2006, http://www.isdscotland.org/isd/info3.jsp?pContentID=1022&p_applic=CCC&p_service=Content.show&.

Jackson, C. and Mander, R. (1995) History or herstory: the decline and fall of the midwife? *British Journal of Midwifery*. 3:5, 279–83.

Jackson, N. and Paterson-Brown, S. (2001) Physical sequelae of caesarean section. *Best Practice and Research in Clinical Obstetrics and Gynaecology*. 15:1, 49–61.

Jakobi, P., Solt, I., Tamir, A. and Zimmer, E.Z. (2002) Over-the-counter oral analgesia for postcesarean pain. *American Journal of Obstetrics and Gynecology*. 187:4, 1066–9.

Johnson, C., Keirse, M., Enkin, M.J.N. and Chalmers, I. (1989) Nutrition and hydration in labour. In Chalmers, I., Enkin, M. and Keirse, M.J.N. (eds), *Effective Care in Pregnancy and Childbirth*. Vol 2. Oxford: Oxford University Press, pp. 827–32.

Johnson, T. (1995) Governmentality and the institutionalisation of expertise. In Johnson, T., Larkin, G. and Saks, M. (eds), *Health Professions and the State in Europe*. London: Routledge, pp. 7–23.

Jordan, M. (2001) Routine surgery: for Brazilian women, caesarean sections are surprisingly popular. *Wall Street Journal*, accessed January 2006, http://www.amigasdoparto.com.br/impr002.html.

Joseph, S. and Bailham, D. (2004) Traumatic childbirth: what we know and what we can do. *Midwives*. 7:6, 258–61.

Jowitt, M. (2001) Problems with RCTs and midwifery. *Midwifery Matters*. 91: Winter, 9–10.

Kasidi, E. (2006) Personal communication.

Kay, M.A. (1982) *Anthropology of Human Birth*. Philadelphia: F.A. Davis Company.

Keirse, M.J.N.C. (2002) In the literature. Evidence-based childbirth only for breech babies? *Birth*. 29:1, 55–9.

Kemppainen, L., Jokelainen, J., Jarvelin, M.R., Isohanni, M. and Rasanen, P. (2001) The one-child family and violent criminality: a 31-year follow-up study of the Northern Finland 1966 Birth Cohort. *American Journal of Psychiatry*. 158, 6960–2.

Kenny, M. (2001) Body politic. Why honeymoon-fresh vaginas are in vogue . . . Caesareans. *Nursing Times*. 97:25, 23.

Khunpradit, S., Lumbiganon, P., Jaipukdee, J. and Laopaiboon, M. (2005) Non-clinical interventions for reducing unnecessary caesarean section. (Protocol) Cochrane Database of Systematic Reviews, Issue 4. Art No CD005528. DOI: 10.1002/14651858.CD005528, accessed January 2006.

King, J.F. (2000) Obstetric interventions among private and public patients: high rates of operative vaginal interventions in private patients need analysis. *British Medical Journal*. 321:7254, 125–6.

Kirby, R.S. and Hanlon-Lundberg, K.M. (1999) Cesarean delivery: improving on Nature? *Birth*. 26:4, 259–62.

Kirkham, M. (1999) The culture of midwifery in the National Health Service in England. *Journal of Advanced Nursing*. 30:3, 732–9.

Kirkham, M.J. (1986) A feminist perspective in midwifery. In Webb, C. (ed.), *Feminist Practice in Women's Health Care*. Chichester: John Wiley.

Kirkham, M. (2000) Choice and bureaucracy. In Kirkham, M.J. (ed.), *Informed Choice in Maternity Care*. Basingstoke: Palgrave Macmillan, Ch. 9.

Kitzinger, J. (1990) Strategies of the early childbirth movement: A case study of the National Childbirth Trust. In Garcia, J., Kilpatrick, R. and Richards, M. (eds), *The Politics of Maternity Care*. Oxford: Clarendon Press.

Kitzinger, S. (1998) The Cesarean Epidemic in Great Britain: Sheila Kitzinger's letter from Europe. *Birth*. 25:1, 56–8.

Kitzinger, S. (2000) *Rediscovering Birth*. London: Little, Brown.

Kitzinger, S. (2005) *The Politics of Birth*. Edinburgh: Elsevier Butterworth Heinemann.

Klaus, M. and Kennell, J. (1982) *Parent Infant Bonding*, 2nd edn. St Louis: Mosby.

Koppel, G.T. and Kaiser, D. (2001) Fathers at the end of their rope: a brief report of fathers abandoned in the perinatal situation. *Journal of Reproductive and Infant Psychology*. 19:3, 249–51.

Koppel, S.M. and Thapar, A. (1998) Treating blood needle phobia. *Hospital Medicine* (London). 59:9, 730–2.

Kotaska, A. (2004) Inappropriate use of randomised trials to evaluate complex phenomena: case study of vaginal breech delivery. *British Medical Journal*. 329:7473, 1039–42.

Kozak, L.J. and Weeks, J.D. (2002) U.S. trends in obstetric procedures, 1990–2000. *Birth*. 29:3, 157–61.

Krupitz, H., Arzt, W., Ebner, T., Sommergruber, M., Steininger, E. and Tews, G. (2005) Assisted vaginal delivery versus caesarean section in breech presentation. *Acta Obstetricia et Gynecologica Scandinavica*. 84:6, 588–92.

Kwast, B.E. (1996) Prolonged and obstructed labour in developing countries: steps to reduce a neglected tragedy. In Murray, S.F. (ed.), *Midwives and Safer Motherhood*. London: Mosby, Ch. 1.

Kwawukume, E.Y. (2001) Caesarean section in developing countries. In Drife, J. and Walker, J. (eds), *Best Practice and Research in Clinical Obstetrics and Gynaecology*. 15:1, 165–78.

Kwee, A., Bots, M.L., Visser, G.H.A. and Bruinse, H.W. (2006) Emergency peripartum hysterectomy: A prospective study in the Netherlands. *European Journal of Obstetrics, Gynecology and Reproductive Biology*. 124:2, 187–92.

Lancet (1985) World Health Organisation: Appropriate Technology for Birth. *The Lancet*. ii:8452, 436–7.

Landon, M.B., Hauth, J.C., Leveno, K.J., Spong, C.Y., Leindecker, S., Varner, M.W., Moawad, A.H., Caritis, S.N., Harper, M., Wapner, R.J., Sorokin, Y., Miodovnik, M., Carpenter, M., Peaceman, A.M., O'Sullivan, M.J., Sibai, B., Langer, O., Thorp, J.M., Ramin, S.M., Mercer, B.M. and Gabbe, S.G. (2004) National Institute of Child Health and Human Development Maternal-Fetal Medicine Units Network. Maternal and perinatal outcomes associated with a trial of labor after prior cesarean delivery. *New England Journal of Medicine*. 351:25, 2581–9.

Lavender, T. (2003) NCT Evidence based briefing – use of the partogram in labour. NCT *New Digest*, 24 September, 14–16.

Lavender, T. and Walkinshaw, S.A. (1998) Can midwives reduce postpartum psychological morbidity? A randomized trial. *Birth*. 25:4, 215–9.

Lavender, T., Wallymahmed, A.H. and Walkinshaw, S.A. (1999) Managing labor using partograms with different action lines: a prospective study of women's views. *Birth*. 26:2, 89–98.

Leboyer, F. (1975) *Birth Without Violence*. New York: Alfred Knopf.

Leeman, L. (2005) Patient-choice cesarean delivery. *American Family Physician*. 72:4, 697, 700, 705.

Leitch, D.B. (1999) Mother–infant interaction: achieving synchrony. *Nursing Research*. 48:1, 55–8.

Lesley, J. (2004) *Birth After Caesarean*. London: AIMS.

Letsky, E.A. (1985) *Haematological Disorders in Pregnancy*. London: W.B. Saunders.

Levitt, R., Wall, A. and Appleby, J. (1995) The reorganised national health service, 5th edn. London: Chapman & Hall.

Lewis, G. (1998) Why Mothers Die 1994–96 – Report on confidential enquiries into maternal deaths in the United Kingdom. London: DoH.

Lewis, G. (2004) Why Mothers Die 2000–2002 – Report on confidential enquiries into maternal deaths in the United Kingdom. London: CEMACH, RCOG.

Lindhard, A., Nielsen, P.V., Mouritsen, L.A., Zachariassen, A., Sorensen, H.U. and Roseno, H. (1990) The implications of introducing the symphyseal-fundal height-measurement. A prospective randomized controlled trial. *British Journal of Obstetrics and Gynaecology*. 97, 675–80.

Lingard, L., Espin, S., Whyte, S., Regehr, G., Baker, G.R., Reznick, R., Bohnen, J., Orser, B., Doran, D. and Grober, E. (2004) Communication failures in the operating room: an observational classification of recurrent types and effects. *Quality and Safety in Health Care*. 135, 330–4.

Liston, W.A. (2003) Rising caesarean section rates: can evolution and ecology explain some of the difficulties of modern childbirth? *Journal of the Royal Society of Medicine*. 96:11, 559–61.

Liu, C., Munakata, T. and Onuoha, F.N. (2005) Mental health condition of the only-child: a study of urban and rural high school students in China. *Adolescence*. 40:160, 831–45.

Llewellyn-Jones, D. (1969) *Fundamentals of Obstetrics and Gynaecology*. London: Faber & Faber.

Lo, J.C. (2003) Patients' attitudes vs. physicians' determination: implications for cesarean sections. *Social Science & Medicine*. 57:1, 91–6.

LoCicero, A.K. (1993) Explaining excessive rates of cesareans and other childbirth interventions: contributions from contemporary theories of gender and psychosocial development. *Social Science & Medicine*. 37:10, 1261–9.

Loeb, M., Main, C., Walker-Dilks, C. and Eady, A. (2003) Antimicrobial drugs for treating methicillin-resistant Staphylococcus aureus colonization. Cochrane Database of Systematic Reviews, Issue 4. Art. No.: CD003340 DOI 10.1002/14651858.CD003340.

Logan, K. (2005) Incontinence and the effects of childbirth on the pelvic floor. *British Journal of Midwifery*. 13:6, 374–7.

Lowdon, G. (1995a) Of No Consequence. NCT New Generation Digest, p. 14.

Lowdon, G. (1995b) Actually. New Generation Digest (National Childbirth Trust) December p. 11, accessed July 2006, http://www.caesarean.org.uk/Articles.html.

Lowdon, G. and Derrick, D.C. (2002) VBAC – on whose terms? *AIMS. Quarterly Journal*. 14:1, 5–7.

Lubic, R.W. (1979) *Barriers and Conflict in Maternity Care Innovation*. New York City: MCA.

Lucas, D.N., Yentis, S.M., Kinsella, S.M., Holdcroft, A., May, A.E., Wee, M. and Robinson, P.N. (2000) Urgency of caesarean section: a new classification. *Journal of Royal Society of Medicine*. 93, 346–50.

Lurie, S. (2005) The changing motives of caesarean section: from the ancient world to the twenty-first century. *Archives of Gynecology and Obstetrics*. 271, 281–5.

Lydon-Rochelle, M.T., Holt, V.L. and Martin, D.P. (2001) Delivery method and self-reported postpartum general health status among primiparous women. *Paediatric and Perinatal Epidemiology*. 15:3, 232–40.

Lydon-Rochelle, M.T., Holt, V.L., Martin, D.P. and Easterling, T.R. (2000) Association between method of delivery and maternal rehospitalization. *JAMA*. 283, 2411–16.

Lyons, G. and Akerman, N. (2005) Problems with general anaesthesia for Caesarean section. *Minerva Anestesiologica*. 71:1–2, 27–38.

MacArthur, C., Glazener, C.M.A., Herbison, P., Wilson, P.D., Lang, D. and Gee, H. (2001) Obstetric practice and faecal incontinence three months after delivery. *British Journal of Obstetrics and Gynaecology*.108:7, 678–83.

McCallum, C. (2005) Explaining caesarean section in Salvador da Bahia, Brazil. *Sociology of Health and Illness*. 27:2, 215–42.

McCandlish, R. (2006) Meeting maternal request for caesarean section – paving the road to hell. *Midwifery*. 22:3, 204–6.

McCourt, C. and Pearce, A. (2000) Does continuity of carer matter to women from minority ethnic groups? *Midwifery*. 16:2, 145–54.

McCrea, B.H. (1996) An investigation of rule-governed behaviours in the control of pain management during the first stage of labour. Unpublished PhD Thesis, University of Ulster.

MacDonald, C., Pinion, S.B. and Macleod, U.M. (2002) Scottish female obstetricians' views on elective caesarean section and personal choice for delivery. *Journal of Obstetrics and Gynaecology*. 22:6, 586–9.

Macfarlane, A.J. (2004) Social class and elective caesareans in the NHS: analysis is not really about social class. *British Medical Journal*. 329:7460, 291.

McGuire, M., Dagge-Bell, F., Purton, P. and Thompson, M. (2004) Shaping maternity services in Scotland. *British Journal of Midwifery*. 12:11, 674–8.

McIlwaine, G., Boulton-Jones, C., Cole, S. and Wilkinson, C. (1998) *Caesarean Section in Scotland 1994/5: a National Audit*. Edinburgh: Scottish Programme for Clinical Effectiveness in Reproductive Health.

McKenna, H.P., Ashton, S. and Keeney, S. (2004) Barriers to evidence-based practice in primary care. *Journal of Advanced Nursing*. 45:2, 178–89.

MacKenzie, I.Z. and Cooke, I.E. (2002) What is a reasonable time from decision to delivery by Caesarean section? Evidence from 533 deliveries. *BJOG: An International Journal of Obstetrics and Gynaecology*. 109, 498–504.

McLeod, C. and Sherwin, S. (2000) Relational autonomy, self-trust, and health care for patients who are oppressed. In Mackenzie, C. and Stoljar, N. (eds), *Relational Autonomy: Feminist Perspective on Autonomy, Agency and the Social Self*. Oxford: Oxford University Press, pp. 259–79.

MacMillan, M. (1994) *Men at Birth*. Royal College of Midwives Survey, London.

Magennis, C., Slevin, E. and Cunningham, J. (1999) Nurses' attitudes to the extension and expansion of their clinical roles. *Nursing Standard*. 13:51, 32–6.

Magill-Cuerden, J. (1997) Comment . . . Whose safety in childbirth? *Modern Midwife*. 7:9, 4–5.

Mahoney, S.F. and Halinka Malcoe, L. (2005) Cesarean delivery in Native American women:

are low rates explained by practices common to the Indian Health Service? *Birth*. 32:3, 170–8.

Mander, R. (1992) See how they learn: Experience as the basis of practice. *Nurse Education Today*. 12:1, 11–18.

Mander, R. (1993a) Epidural analgesia 1: recent history. *British Journal of Midwifery*. 1:6, 259–64.

Mander, R. (1993b) 'Who chooses the choices?' *Modern Midwife*. 3:1, 23–5.

Mander, R. (1995a) *The Care of the Mother Grieving a Baby Relinquished for Adoption*. Aldershot: Avebury.

Mander, R. (1995b) The relevance of the Dutch system of maternity care to the United Kingdom. *Journal of Advanced Nursing*. 22:6, 1023–6.

Mander, R. (1996a) Needs must: publication and the midwife. *British Journal of Midwifery*. 4:2, 77–8.

Mander, R. (1996b) The childfree midwife: the significance of personal experience of childbearing. *Midwives* 109:1302, 186–8.

Mander, R. (1997) Choosing the choices in the USA: examples in the maternity area. *Journal of Advanced Nursing*. 25:6, 1192–7.

Mander, R. (1998) Analgesia and anaesthesia in childbirth: obscurantism and obfuscation. *Journal of Advanced Nursing* 28:1, 86–93.

Mander, R. (1999) Research in midwifery. In Bennett, R. and Brown, L. (eds), *Myles Textbook for Midwives*, 13th edn. Edinburgh: Churchill Livingstone.

Mander, R. (2001a) *Supportive Care and Midwifery*. Oxford: Blackwell Science.

Mander, R. (2001b) Death of a mother: taboo and the midwife. *Practising Midwife*. 4:8, 23–5.

Mander, R. (2001c) The midwife's ultimate paradox: a UK-based study of the death of a mother. *Midwifery*. 17:4, 248–59.

Mander, R. (2004a) *Men and Maternity*. London: Routledge.

Mander, R. (2004b) Little Emperors? Nursing Studies Newsletter, University of Edinburgh, June, p. 2.

Mander, R. (2006a) From 'steering' to partnership. *Journal of Advanced Nursing*. 53:1, 122–3.

Mander, R. (2006b) *Loss and Bereavement in Childbearing*, 2nd edn. London: Routledge.

Mander, R. (In press) Between a rock and a hard place: the situation of the Finnish Midwife. In Reid, L. (ed.), *Freedom to Practise*. London: Routledge.

Mangesi, L. and Hofmeyr, G.J. (2002) Early compared with delayed oral fluids and food after caesarean section. Cochrane Database of Systematic Reviews, Issue 3. Art. No.: CD003516. DOI: 10.1002/14651858.CD003516.

Marks, C., Fethers, K. and Mindel, A. (1999) Management of women with recurrent genital herpes in pregnancy in Australia. *Sexually Transmitted Infections*. 75:1, 55–7.

Marland, H. (1993) The '*burgerlijke*' midwife; the '*stadsvroedvrouw*' of eighteenth-century Holland. In Marland, H. (ed.), *The Art of Midwifery: Early Modern Midwives in Europe*. London: Routledge, pp. 192–213.

Marshall, R.K. (1983) *Virgins and Viragos: A History of Women in Scotland From 1080 to 1980*. London: Collins.

Mason, J. (2000) Letter: Midwives 'verging on the sadistic'. *British Journal of Midwifery*. 8:4, 247.

Mathai, M. and Hofmeyr, G.J. (2003) Abdominal surgical incisions for caesarean section. (Protocol) Cochrane Database of Systematic Reviews, Issue 4. Art. No.: CD004453. DOI: 10.1002/14651858.CD004453.

Maymon, R., Halperin, R., Mendlovic, S., Schneider, D. and Herman, A. (2004) Ectopic pregnancies in a Caesarean scar: review of the medical approach to an iatrogenic complication. *Human Reproduction* Update. 10:6, 515–23.

Maynard, S.E., Venkatesha, S., Thadhani, R. and Karumanchi, S.A. (2005) Soluble Fms-like tyrosine kinase 1 and endothelial dysfunction in the pathogenesis of pre-eclampsia. *Pediatric Research*. 57:5 Pt 2, 1R–7R.

Meier, P.R. and Porreco, R.P. (1982) Trial of labour following caesarean section: a two year experience. *American Journal of Obstetrics and Gynecology*. 144:6, 671–8.

Meikle, S.F., Steiner, C.A., Zhang, J. and Lawrence, W.L. (2005) A national estimate of the elective primary cesarean delivery rate. *Obstetrics and Gynecology*. 105, 751–6.

Melia, K.M. (2004) *Health Care Ethics: Lessons From Intensive Care*. London: Sage.

Menacker, F. (2005) Trends in Cesarean Rates for First Births and Repeat Cesarean Rates for Low-Risk Women: United States, 1990–2003. National Vital Statistics Reports 54:4, September 22, accessed March 2006, http://www.cdc.gov/nchs/.

Menage, J. (1993) Post-traumatic stress disorder in women who have undergone obstetric and/or gynaecological procedures. *Journal of Reproductive and Infant Psychology*. 11:4, 221–8.

Mendelson, C.L. (1946) The aspiration of stomach contents into the lungs during obstetric anesthesia. *American Journal of Obstetrics and Gynecology*. 52, 191–205.

Menken, J. and Rahman, O. (2001) Reproductive health. In Merson, M.H., Black, R.E. and Mills, A.J. (eds), *International Public Health: Diseases, Programs, Systems, and Policies*. Gaithersburg, MD: Aspen.

Miller, D.A., Rabello, Y.A. and Paul, R.H. (1996) The modified biophysical profile: antepartum testing in the 1990s. *American Journal of Obstetrics and Gynecology*. 174:3, 812–17.

Miller, J.M. Jr (1988) Maternal and neonatal morbidity and mortality in cesarean section. *Obstetrical and Gynecological Clinics of North America*. 15, 629–38.

Milner, A.D., Saunders, R.A. and Hopkin, I.E. (1978) Effects of delivery by caesarean section on lung mechanics and lung volume in the human neonate. *Archives of Disease in Childhood*. 53:7, 545–8.

Moes, C.B. and Thacher, F. (2001) The midwife as first assistant for cesarean section. *Journal of Midwifery and Women's Health*. 46:5 305–12.

Moir-Bussy, B.R., Hulton, R.M. and Thompson, J.R. (1985) Wound infection after Caesarean section. *Journal of Hospital Infection*. 5, 359–70.

Mollison, J., Porter, M., Campbell, D. and Bhattacharyab, S. (2005) Primary mode of delivery and subsequent pregnancy. *BJOG: An International Journal of Obstetrics and Gynaecology*. 112:8, 1061–5.

Mossialos, E., Allin, S., Karras, K. and Davaki, K. (2005) An investigation of Caesarean sections in three Greek hospitals: the impact of financial incentives and convenience. *European Journal of Public Health*. 15:3, 288–95.

Moyzakitis, W. (2004) Exploring women's descriptions of distress and/or trauma of childbirth from a feminist perspective. *RCM Evidence Based Midwifery*. 2:1, 8–14.

Mozurkewich, E.L. and Hutton, E.K. (2000) Elective repeat cesarean delivery versus trial of labor: a meta-analysis of the literature from 1989 to 1999. *American Journal of Obstetrics and Gynecology*. 183:5, 1187–97.

Murphy, D.J., Stirrat, G.M. and Heron, J. (2002) ALSPAC Study Team. The relationship between Caesarean section and subfertility in a population-based sample of 14 541 pregnancies. *Human Reproduction*. 17:7, 1914–17.

Murphy-Black, T. (1990) Introduction. In Faulkner, A. and Murphy-Black, T. (eds), *Midwifery: Excellence In Nursing – The Research Route*. London: Scutari.

NCT (National Childbirth Trust) (2003) NCT calls for better birthing facilities: poor birth environments could reduce 'normal' births. *Practising Midwife*. 6:7, 8.

Neilson, J.P. (2003) Fetal electrocardiogram (ECG) for fetal monitoring during labour. Cochrane Database of Systematic Reviews, Issue 2. Art. No.: CD000116. DOI: 10.1002/14651858.CD000116.

Newell, M.L. (2006) Current issues in the prevention of mother-to-child transmission of HIV-1 infection. *Transactions of the Royal Society of Tropical Medicine and Hygiene*. 100:1, 1–5.

Newman, R. (1998) Obstetric management of higher order multiple pregnancies. *Baillière's Clinical Obstetrics and Gynaecology*. 12, 109–27.

NICE (2004) Caesarean Section, Clinical Guideline. National Collaborating Centre for Women's and Children's Health National Institute for Clinical Excellence.

Nice, C., Feeney, A., Godwin, P., Mohanraj, M., Edwards, A., Baldwin, A., Choyce, A., Hunt, A., Kinnaird, C., Maloney, M., Anderson, W. and Campbell, L. (1996) A prospective audit of wound infection rates after caesarean section in five West Yorkshire hospitals. *Journal of Hospital Infection*. 33:1, 55–61.

Nicoll, A.E., Black, C., Powls, A. and Mackenzie, F. (2003) An audit of neonatal respiratory morbidity following elective caesarean section at term. *Scottish Medical Journal*. 49:1, 22–5.

Nightingale, F. (1859) *Notes On Nursing: What It Is, And What It Is Not*. London: Harrison,.

Nightingale, F. (1863) Correspondence relating to the Crimea, India and Public Health Reform, London, The British Library, accessed December 2005, http://www.adam-matthew-publications.co.uk/collections_az/Nightingale-1/description.aspx.

Nikolajsen, L., Sorensen, H.C., Jensen, T.S. and Kehlet, H. (2004) Chronic pain following caesarean section. *Acta Anaesthesiologica Scandinavica*. 48:1, 111–16.

Nikolentzos, A. (2005) Can existing theories of Professions, Institutions and Medical Power explain the Greek health care reforms since 1983? Accessed March 2006, http://www.lse.ac.uk/collections/hellenicObservatory/events/2ndPhDSymposium_June2005/symposiumPapersOnline05.htm#generated-subheading1.

NTUH (2005) Cesarean section: a brief history. National Taipei University Hospital, accessed December 2005, http://memo.cgu.edu.tw/%C1%C2%C0%E9%B0%F3/history.htm.

Nuland, S.B. (2004) Mistakes in the operating room – error and responsibility. *New England Journal of Medicine*. 351:13, 1281–3.

Nuttall, C. (2000) Caesarean section controversy. The caesarean culture of Brazil. *British Medical Journal*. 320:7241, 1074.

NWPH (2005) Births Data North West Public Health, accessed March 2006, www.nwph.net/nwpho/inequalities/ health_wealth_ch21_(2).pdf.

O'Brien-Abel, N. (2003) Uterine rupture during VBAC trial of labour: risk factors and fetal response. *Journal of Midwifery and Women's Health*. Online July/Aug 48:4.

O'Driscoll, K. and Meagher, D. (1986) *Active Management of Labour*, 2nd edn. London: Baillière Tindall.

O'Driscoll, K., Meagher, D. and Boylan, P. (1993) *Active Management of Labour: The Dublin Experience*, 3rd edn. London: Mosby.

O'Driscoll, K., Meagher, D. and Robson, M. (2003) *Active Management of Labour*, 4th edn. St Louis: Mosby.

OAA/AAGBI (2005) Guidelines for Obstetric Anaesthetic Services Association of

Anaesthetists of Great Britain and Ireland/Obstetric Anaesthetists' Association, accessed May 2006, www.aagbi.org/pdf/Obstetric.pdf.

Oakley, A. (1983) Social consequences of obstetric technology: the importance of measuring 'soft' outcomes. *Birth*. 10:2, 99–108.

Oakley, A. (1993) The follow-up survey. In Chamberlain, G., Wraight, A. and Steer, P. (eds), *Pain and Its Relief In Childbirth: The Results of a National Survey Conducted by the National Birthday Trust*. Edinburgh: Churchill Livingstone, ch. 10.

Oakley, A. and Richards, M.P.M. (1990) Caesarean deliveries. In Garcia, J., Kilpatrick, R. and Richards, M. (eds), *The Politics of Maternity Care*. Oxford: Clarendon Press, ch. 10.

Odent, M. (1987) The fetus ejection reflex. *Birth*. 14:2, 104–5.

Odent, M. (1993) *The Nature of Birth and Breastfeeeding*. Westport: Bergin & Garvey.

Odent, M. (2004) *The Caesarean*. London: Free Association.

OECD (2003) OECD Health Data, Infant mortality rate. Accessed March 2006, http://www.oecd.org/document/16/0,2340,en_2825_495642_20852001111,00.html.

OECD (2005) Health and spending resources, accessed March 2006, http://www.oecd.org/topicstatsportal/0,2647,en_2825_49564211111,00.html.

Ogilvie, H. (1948) Large intestine colic due to sympathetic deprivation: a new clinical syndrome. *British Medical Journal*. 2, 671–3.

Olufowobi, O., Sorinola, O., Miller, S.J. and Condie, R.G. (2003) Scar endometrioma: a cause for concern in the light of the rising caesarean section rate. *Journal of Obstetrics & Gynaecology*. 23:1, 86.

Orasanu, J. and Connolly, T. (1993) The reinvention of decision making. In Klein, G., Orasanu, J., Calderwood, R. and Zsambok, C. (eds), *Decision Making in Action. Models and Methods*. Norwood, NJ: Ablex Publishing Corporation, pp. 3–20.

Osterman, J.E., Hopper, J.W., Heran, W.J., Keane, T.M. and Van der Kolk, B.A. (2001) Awareness under anesthesia and development of posttraumatic stress disorder. *General Hospital Psychiatry*. 23:4, 198–204.

Padmadas, S.S., Kumar, S.S., Nair, S.B. and Kumari, A. (2000) Caesarean section delivery in Kerala, India: evidence from a national family health survey. *Social Science & Medicine*. 51:4, 511–21.

Page, G., Buntinx, F. and Hanssens, M. (2003) Indwelling bladder catheterization as part of postoperative care for caesarean section. (Protocol) Cochrane Database of Systematic Reviews, Issue 3. Art. No.: CD004354. DOI: 10.1002/14651858.CD004354.

Paranjothy, S., Liu, E., Brown, H. and Thomas, J. (2004) Drugs at caesarean section for preventing nausea, vomiting and aspiration pneumonitis. (Protocol) Cochrane Database of Systematic Reviews, Issue 4. Art. No.: CD004943. DOI: 10.1002/14651858.CD004943.

Parsons, M. (2004) A midwifery practice dichotomy on oral intake in labour. *Midwifery*. 20:1, 72–81.

Patel, R.R., Murphy, D.J. and Peters, T.J. (2005) Operative delivery and postnatal depression: a cohort study. *British Medical Journal*. 330:7496, 879.

Paterson-Brown, S. (1998) Should doctors perform an elective caesarean section on request? Yes, as long as the woman is fully informed. *British Medical Journal*. 317:7156, 462–3.

Pearce, E.M. and Dodd, J.M. (2004) Rectal analgesia for pain relief after caesarean section. (Protocol) Cochrane Database of Systematic Reviews, Issue 2. Art. No.: CD004738. DOI: 10.1002/14651858.CD004738.

Penn, R.G. (1986) Iatrogenic disease: an historical survey of adverse reactions before thalidomide. In D'Arcy, P.F. and Griffin, J.P. (eds), *Iatrogenic Diseases*, 3rd edn. Oxford: Oxford University Press, p. 14.

Penn, Z. and Ghaem-Maghami, S. (2001) Indications for caesarean section. *Best Practice and Research Clinical Obstetrics and Gynaecology*. 15:1, 1–15.

Petrou, S., Henderson, J. and Glazener, C. (2001) Economic aspects of caesarean section and alternative modes of delivery. *Best Practice and Research in Clinical Obstetrics and Gynaecology*. 15:1, 145–63.

Philpott, R.H. (1972) Graphic records in labour. *British Medical Journal*. 4:833, 163–5.

Plati, C., Lemonidou, C., Katostaras, T., Mantas, J. and Lanara, V. (1998) Nursing manpower development and strategic planning in Greece. *Image: Journal of Nursing Scholarship*. 30:4, 329–33.

Pollock, A. and Price, D. (2000) Globalisation? Privatisation! *Healthmatters*. 41, Summer, 12–13.

Porter, M., Bhattacharya, S., Van Teijlingen, E. and Templeton, A. for the Reproductive Outcome Following Caesarean Section (ROCS) Collaborative Group (2003) Does Caesarean section cause infertility? *Human Reproduction*. 18:10, 1983–6.

Potter, J.E., Berquo, E., Perpetuo, I.H., Leal, O.F., Hopkins, K., Souza, M.R. and Formiga, M.C. (2001) Unwanted caesarean sections among public and private patients in Brazil: prospective study. *British Medical Journal*. 323:7322, 1155–8.

Pratten, B. (1990) *Power, Politics and Pregnancy*. London: Health Rights.

Princeton (2005) Wordnet, accessed November 2005, http://wordnet.princeton.edu/perl/webwn?s=caesarean.

Propper, C. (2001) Expenditure on Health Care in the UK: A review of the issues. Department of Economics and CMPO University of Bristol, CASE LSE and CEPR. Accessed March 2006, www.bris.ac.uk/cmpo/workingpapers/wp30.pdf.

Quecke, K. (1952) Über die Anfänge des Kaiserschnittes [About the origins of the caesarean]. Ciba-Zeitschrift (ed.), *Der Kaiserschnitt*. 128, 4706–11.

Ramsay, B. and Paine, P. (1997) Assisting at caesarean section: another role of the midwife? *MIDIRS Midwifery Digest*. 7:4, 481–2.

RCM (1995) RCM Survey – 'Men at Birth'. *Midwives*. 108:1284, 18.

RCOG (1995) *Working party report on prophylaxis against thromboembolism in Gynaecology and Obstetrics*. London: RCOG.

RCOG (2006) ECV and reducing the incidence of breech presentation. London Royal College of Obstetricians and Gynaecologists. Accessed April 2006, http://www.rcog.org.uk/index.asp?pageID=23.

RCSE (2003) Factors Affecting Wound Healing, accessed February 2006, http://www.edu.rcsed.ac.uk/Wound%20Management/Factors%20Affecting%20Wound%20Healing.htm.

RCSE (2006) Wound Healing, accessed July 2006, http://www.edu.rcsed.ac.uk/Wound%20Management/Factors%20Affecting%20Wound%20Healing.htm.

Rees, C. (1997) *An Introduction to Research for Midwives*. Hale: Books for Midwives.

Revill, J. (2006) Why mothers should be offered caesareans. *Observer*. 05.03.06.

Richards, M.P.M. (1982) The trouble with choice in childbirth. *Birth*. 9:4, 253–60.

Ridley, R.T., Davis, P.A., Bright, J.H. and Sinclair, D. (2002) What influences a woman to choose vaginal birth after cesarean? *JOGNN: Journal of Obstetric, Gynecologic, and Neonatal Nursing*. 31:6, 665–72.

Roberts, C.L., Tracy, S. and Peat, B. (2000) Rates for obstetric intervention among private and public patients in Australia: population based descriptive study. *British Medical Journal*. 321, 137–41.

Roberts, C.L., Algert, C.S., Carnegie, M. and Peat, B. (2002) Operative delivery during labour: trends and predictive factors. *Paediatric and Perinatal Epidemiology*. 16:2, 115–23.

Robertson, A. (2003) Andrea's Diary October 18, Unethical Caesarean research. Accessed December 2005, http://birthinternational.co.uk/diary/archives/cat_midwifery.html.

Robertson, A. (2004) Letter from Oz. *MIDIRS Midwifery Digest*. 14:1, 132–3.

Robinson, E.J., Kerr, C., Stevens, A., Lilford, R., Braunholtz, D., Edwards, S. (2004) Lay conceptions of the ethical and scientific justifications for random allocation in clinical trials. *Social Science & Medicine*. 58:4, 811–24.

Robinson, J. (2000) Consumer comments. Richer women, worse care? *British Journal of Midwifery*. 8:5, 280.

Robinson, J. (2002) Emergency caesareans – how long does it take? *AIMS Journal*. 14:1, 17–18.

Robinson, J. (2002/03) Female obstetricians choose vaginal birth. *AIMS Journal*. 14:4, 13–14.

Robinson, J. (2005) Ethics watch. *AIMS Journal*. 17:2, 3–5.

Romney, M. (1980) Predelivery shaving: an unjustified assault? *Journal of Obstetrics & Gynaecology*. 1, 33–5.

Rosenberg, K. and Trevathan, W. (2002) Birth, obstetrics and human evolution. *British Journal of Obstetrics and Gynaecology*. 109:11, 1199–206.

Rosser, J. (1994) World Health Organisation Partograph in management of labour. *MIDIRS Midwifery Digest*. 4:4, 436–7.

Rothwell, H. (1996) Changing childbirth . . . changing nothing. *Midwives*. 109:1306, 291–4.

Ryan, J.G. (2002) The chapel and the operating room: the struggle of Roman Catholic clergy, physicians, and believers with the dilemmas of obstetric surgery, 1800–1900. *Bulletin of the History of Medicine*. 76:3, 461–94.

Ryding, E.L., Wijma, K. and Wijma, B. (1998) Experiences of emergency cesarean section: A phenomenological study of 53 women. *Birth*. 25:4, 246–51.

Ryding, E.L., Persson, A., Onell, C. and Kvist, L. (2003) An evaluation of midwives' counseling of pregnant women in fear of childbirth. *Acta Obstetricia et Gynecologica Scandinavica*. 82:1, 10–17.

Sackett, D., Rosenburg, W., Gray, J.A., Haynes, B. and Richardson, W.S. (1996) Evidence based medicine: what it is and what it isn't. *British Medical Journal*. 312:7023, 71–2.

Saddam, Hussein (1991) 'The Mother of All Battles Begins'. Accessed January 2006, http://news.bbc.co.uk/onthisday/hi/dates/stories/january/17/newsid_2530000/2530375.stm.

Savage, W. (1986) *A Savage Enquiry: Who Controls Childbirth?* London: Virago.

SCC (Scottish Consumer Council) (2001) *Access to Primary Care Services in Scotland*. Edinburgh: Scottish Executive Health Department.

SCoH (2003) Written Evidence Select Committee on Health HoC. Accessed July 2006, http://www.publications.parliament.uk/pa/cm200203/cmselect/cmhealth/796/796we06.htm.

Scott, R. (2000) The pregnant woman and the good Samaritan: can a woman have a duty to undergo a caesarean section? *Oxford Journal of Legal Studies*. 20:3, 407–36.

Scully, D. (1994) *Men Who Control Women's Health: The Miseducation of Obstetrician-Gynecologists*. New York: Teachers College Press.

SE (2006) Healthcare associated infection. Scottish Executive, accessed 2 June 2006, http://www.scotland.gov.uk/Topics/Health/NHS-Scotland/19529/cnotips.

Sehdev, H.M. (2005) Cesarean delivery. Accessed 19 December 2005, http://www.emedicine.com/med/topic3283.htm.

Semprini, A.B., Castagna, C., Ravizza, M., Fiore, S., Savasi, V., Muggiasca, M.L., Grossi, E., Guerra, B., Tibaldi, C. and Scaravelli, G. (1995) The incidence of complications after caesarean section in 156 HIV-positive women. *AIDS*. 9:8, 913–17.

Sharpe, V.A. and Faden, A.I. (1998) *Medical Harm: Historical, Conceptual, and Ethical Dimensions of Iatrogenic Illness*. Cambridge: Cambridge University Press.

Sheahan, D. (1972) The game of the name, nurse professional and nurse technician. *Nursing Outlook*. 20, 440–4.

SHSSC (2000) Women's Voices: Women's Experiences of Maternity Services at Craigavon Area Hospital following Transfer from South Tyrone Hospital, June. Southern Health and Social Services Council.

Simkin, P. and Ancheta, R. (2000) *The Labour Progress Handbook*. Oxford: Blackwell Science.

Sjögren, B. (1998) Fear of childbirth and psychosomatic support. *Acta Obstetrica et Gynecologica Scandinavica*. 77:3, 819–25.

Skippen, M., Kirkup, J., Maxton, R.M. and Mcdonald, S.W. (2004) The chain saw – a Scottish invention. *Scottish Medical Journal*. 49:2, 57–60.

Sleep, J., Grant, A., Garcia, J., Elbourne, D., Spencer, J. and Chalmers, I. (1984) West Berkshire perineal management trial. *British Medical Journal Clinical Research*. 289:6445, 587–90.

Slome, J. (2002) A midwife's private practice in Israel. *British Journal of Midwifery*. 10:4, 224–9.

Smaill, F. and Hofmeyr, G.J. (2002) Antibiotic prophylaxis for cesarean section. Cochrane Database of Systematic Reviews, Issue 3. Art. No.: CD000933. DOI: 10. 1002/14651858. CD000933.

Small, R., Lumley, J., Donohue, L., Potter, A. and Waldenström, U. (2000) Randomised controlled trial of midwife led debriefing to reduce maternal depression after operative childbirth. *British Medical Journal*. 321:7268, 1043–7.

Smellie, W. (1752) *A Treatise on the Theory and Practice of Midwifery*. London, printed for D. Wilson.

Smit, Y., Scherjon, S.A. and Treffers, P.E. (1997) Elderly nulliparae in midwifery care in Amsterdam. *Midwifery*. 13:2, 73–7.

Smith, G.C.S., Pell, J.P. and Dobbie, R. (2002) Birth order, gestational age, and risk of delivery related perinatal death in twins: retrospective cohort study. *British Medical Journal*. 325:7371, 1004.

Smith, G.D. (2006) Personal communication.

Smith, J.F., Hernandez, C. and Wax, J.R. (1997) Fetal laceration injury at cesarean delivery. *Obstetrics and Gynecology*. 90:3, 344–6.

SOS (2002) Survivors of symphysiotomy, accessed 19 December 2005, http://www.bbc.co.uk/radio4/womanshour/2002_50_mon_01.shtml.

SPCERH (2001) *Expert Advisory Group on Caesarean Section in Scotland*. Edinburgh: SPCERH.

SPCERH (2005) *NHS Board Variations in Maternity Care Outcomes*. Edinburgh: Scottish Programme for Clinical Effectiveness in Reproductive Health.

Stanton, C.K., Dubourg, D., De Brouwere, V., Pujades, M. and Ronsmans, C. (2005) Reliability of data on caesarean sections in developing countries. *Bulletin of the World Health Organization*. 83:6, 449–55.

Stapleton, H. (2004) Is there a difference between a free gift and a planned purchase? The use of evidence-based leaflets in maternity care. In Kirkham, M.J. (ed.), *Informed Choice in Maternity Care*. Basingstoke: Palgrave Macmillan, p. 87.

Stapleton, H., Kirkham, M. and Thomas, G. (2002) Qualitative study of evidence based leaflets in maternity care. *British Medical Journal*. 324:7338, 639–44.

Steele, A.M. and Beadle, M. (2003) A survey of postnatal debriefing. *Journal of Advanced Nursing*. 43:21,30–6.

Steer, P. (1998) Caesarean section: an evolving procedure? *British Journal of Obstetrics and Gynaecology*. 105:10, 1052–5.

Stephens, L. (1998) Male power: a challenge to normal childbirth. *British Journal of Midwifery*. 6:7, 450–3.

Sterne, L. (1769) *The Life and Opinions of Tristram Shandy, Gentleman*. London: Dodslett.

Stewart, S. (2001) The use of internet resources by midwives in New Zealand. Unpublished MA Thesis, Victoria University of Wellington.

Stewart, S. (2005) Caught in the web: an over view of e-health and midwifery practice. *British Journal of Midwifery*. 13:9, 546–50.

Sultan, A. and Stanton, S. (1996) Preserving the pelvic floor and perineum during childbirth – elective caesarean section? *British Journal of Obstetrics and Gynaecology*. 103, 731–4.

Sultan, A.H., Kamm, M.A., Hudson, C.N. and Thomas Bartram, C.I. (1993) Anal sphincter disruption during vaginal delivery. *New England Journal of Medicine*. 329, 1905–11.

Symon, A. (2000a) Litigation and defensive clinical practice: quantifying the problem. *Midwifery*. 16:1, 8–14.

Symon, A. (2000b) Litigation and changes in professional behaviour: a qualitative appraisal. *Midwifery*. 16:1, 15–21.

Tague, R.G. and Lovejoy, C.O. (1986) The obstetric pelvis of A.L.288-1 (Lucy). *Journal of Human Evolution*. 15, 237–73.

Tanner, J., Woodings, D. and Moncaster, K. (2003) Pre-operative hair removal to reduce surgical site infection. (Protocol) The Cochrane Database of Systematic Reviews, Issue 2. Art. No.: CD004122. DOI: 10.1002/14651858.CD004122.

Taylor, L.K., Simpson, J.M., Roberts, C.L., Olive, E.C. and Henderson-Smart, D.J. (2005) Risk of complications in a second pregnancy following caesarean section in the first pregnancy: a population-based study. *Medical Journal of Australia*. 183:10, 515–9.

TBT (2004) Information about the Term Breech Trial News 10:1, p. 1. Accessed August 2006, http://www.utoronto.ca/miru/breech/index_tbt.htm?/miru/breech/tbt.htm.

Tempest, M. (2006) Labour counters Cameron's pitch to parents. *Guardian* Society, June 20.

Tenon, J.R. (1788) *Mémoires sur les hôpitaux de Paris*. Paris: De l'imprimerie de Ph. D. Pierres.

Thacker, S.B., Stroup, D. and Chang, M. (2001) Continuous electronic heart rate monitoring for fetal assessment during labor. Cochrane Database of Systematic Reviews, Issue 2. Art. No.: CD000063. DOI: 10.1002/14651858.CD000063.

Thomas, J. and Paranjothy, S. (2001) Royal College of Obstetricians and Gynaecologists Audit Report. RCOG Press Clinical Effectiveness Support Unit. National Sentinel Caesarean Section.

Thomas, P. (2000) Hospital-acquired infections turning birth into an illness. *AIMS Journal*. 12:3, 5–6.

Thompson, I.E., Melia, K.M., Boyd, K.M. and Horsburgh, D. (2006) *Nursing Ethics*, 5th edn. Edinburgh: Churchill Livingstone.

Thompson, J.F., Roberts, C.L., Currie, M. and Ellwood, D.A. (2002) Prevalence and persistence of health problems after childbirth: associations with parity and method of birth. *Birth*. 29:2, 83–94.

Trimbos, J.B. and Keirse, M.J.N.C. (1978) Observer variability in assessment of antepartum cardiotocograms. *British Journal of Obstetrics and Gynaecology*. 85, 900–6.

Trolle, D. (1982) *The History of Caesarean Section.* Copenhagen: Reitzel.

Tucker, J., Hundley, V., Kiger, A., Bryers, H., Caldow, J., Farmer, J., Harris, F., Ireland, J. and van Teijlingen, E. (2005) Sustainable maternity services in remote and rural Scotland? A qualitative survey of staff views on required skills, competencies and training. *Quality and Safety in Health Care.* 14:1, 34–40.

Tussing, A.D. and Wojtowycz, M.A. (1997) Malpractice, defensive medicine, and obstetric behavior. *Medical Care.* 35, 2172–91.

UNPF (2006) O Renew: The Campaign to end fistula. United Nations Population Fund. Accessed July 2006, http://www.endfistula.org/index.htm.

Uotila, J., Tuimala, R. and Kirkinen, P. (2005) Good perinatal outcome in selective vaginal breech delivery at term. *Acta Obstetricia et Gynecologica Scandinavica.* 84:6, 578–83.

Van De Velde, M. (2000) What is the best way to provide postoperative pain therapy after caesarean section? *Current Opinion in Anaesthesiology.* 13, 267–70.

Varner, M.W., Fraser, A.M., Hunter, C.Y., Corneli, P.S. and Ward, R.H. (1996) The intergenerational predisposition to operative delivery. *Obstetrics and Gynecology.* 87:6, 905–11.

Varney Burst, H. (1983) The influence of consumers in the birthing movement. *Topics in Clinical Nursing.* 5, 42–54.

Wagner, M. (2000) Choosing caesarean section. *Lancet.* 356:9242, 1677–80.

Wagner, M. (2002) Critique of the British RCOG National Sentinel Caesarean Section Audit report of Oct 2001. *MIDIRS Midwifery Digest.* 12:3, 366–70.

Waldenström, U. (2004) Why do some women change their opinion about childbirth over time? *Birth.* 31:2, 102–7.

Walker, R., Turnbull, D. and Wilkinson, C. (2004) Increasing cesarean section rates: exploring the role of culture in an Australian community. *Birth.* 31:2, 117–24.

Walt, G. (1998) Globalisation of international health. *Lancet.* 351:9100, 434–7.

Warwick, C. (2001) A midwifery perception of the rising caesarean rate. *MIDIRS Midwifery Digest.* 11:2, 152–6.

Wax, J.R., Cartin, A., Pinette, M.G. and Blackstone, J. (2004) Patient choice cesarean: an evidence-based review. *Obstetrical and Gynecological Survey.* 59:8, 601–16.

Weaver, J. (2000) Talking about caesarean section. *MIDIRS Midwifery Digest.* 10:4, 487–90.

Weaver, J. (2004) Caesarean section and maternal choices. *Fetal and Maternal Medicine Review.* 15:1, 1–25.

Weaver, J.J. and Statham, H. (2005) Wanting a caesarean section: the decision process. *British Journal of Midwifery.* 13:6, 370–3.

Wenger, D.R. (2000) Lexicon of orthopaedic etymology. *Journal of Pediatric Orthopedics.* 20:2, 276.

Westert, G.P., Smits, J.P., Polder, J.J. and Mackenbach, J.P. (2003) Community income and surgical rates in the Netherlands. *Journal of Epidemiology and Community Health.* 57:7, 519–22.

WHO (1994) World Health Organization partograph in management of labour. *Lancet.* 343:8910, 1399–404. World Health Organization maternal health and safe motherhood programme.

WHO (1998) Gender and Health: A Technical Paper: Geneva World Health Organisation. Accessed February 2006, http://www.who.int/reproductive-health/publications/WHD_98_16_gender_and_health_technical_paper/WHD_98_16_table_of_contents_en.html.

WHO (2005) Country Health Indicators, accessed March 2006, http://www3.who.int/whosis/country/indicators.cfm?country=gbr.

WHO (2006) World Health Organisation Country Guide, accessed February 2006, http://www.who.int/countries/en/.

Whyte, H., Hannah, M.E., Saigal, S., Hannah, W.J., Hewson, S., Amankwah, K., Cheng, M., Gafni, A., Guselle, P., Helewa, M., Hodnett, E.D., Hutton, E., Kung, R., McKay, D., Ross, S. and Willan, A. (2004) Term Breech Trial Collaborative Group. Outcomes of children at 2 years after planned cesarean birth versus planned vaginal birth for breech presentation at term: the International Randomized Term Breech Trial. *American Journal of Obstetrics and Gynecology*. 191:3, 864–71.

Wickham, S. (2002) *What's Right For Me? Making Decisions in Pregnancy and Birth.* AIMS: London.

Wiggins, M. and Newburn, M. (2004) Information used by pregnant women. In Kirkham, M. (ed.), *Informed Choice in Maternity Care.* Basingstoke: Macmillan Palgrave, p. 147.

Wilkinson, A.B. and Norrie, K.McK. (1993) *The Law Relating to Parent and Child in Scotland.* Edinburgh: W. Green/Sweet & Maxwell.

Williams, Z. (2005) A fertile gesture. *Guardian*, October 1.

Willson, H. (2000) Factors affecting the administration of analgesia to patients following repair of a fractured hip. *Journal of Advanced Nursing*. 31:5, 1145–54.

Wilson, A.C., Forsyth, J.S., Greene, S.A., Irvine, L., Hau, C. and Howie, P.W. (1998) Relation of infant diet to childhood health: seven year follow up of cohort of children in Dundee infant feeding study. *British Medical Journal*. 316:7124, 21–5.

Wiysonge, C.S., Shey, M.S., Shang, J.D., Sterne, J.A.C. and Brocklehurst, P. (2005) Vaginal disinfection for preventing mother-to-child transmission of HIV infection. Cochrane Database of Systematic Reviews, Issue 4. Art. No.: CD003651. DOI: 10.1002/14651858. CD003651.pub2.

Wrightson, P. (1996) Incidence of infection after Caesarean section: a study. *Nursing Standard*. 10:37. 34–7.

Wykes, C.B., Johnston, T.A., Paterson-Brown, S. and Johanson, R.B. (2003) Symphysiotomy: a lifesaving procedure. *BJOG: An International Journal of Obstetrics and Gynaecology.* 110:2, 219.

Zaki, Z.M.S., Bahar, A.M., Ali, M.E., Albar, H.A.M. and Gerais, M.A. (1998) Risk factors and morbidity in patients with placenta previa accreta compared to placenta previa non-accreta. *Acta Obstetricia et Gynecologica Scandinavica*. 77:4, 391–4.

Zhang, J., Troendle, J.F. and Yancey, M.K. (2002) Reassessing the labor curve in nulliparous women. *American Journal of Obstetrics and Gynecology*. 187:4, 824–8.

Ziadeh, S.M. and Sunna, E.I. (1995) Decreased cesarean birth rates and improved perinatal outcome: a seven-year study. *Birth*. 22:3, 144–7.

Index